IMAGES
of America

MIDDLE TENNESSEE HORSE BREEDING

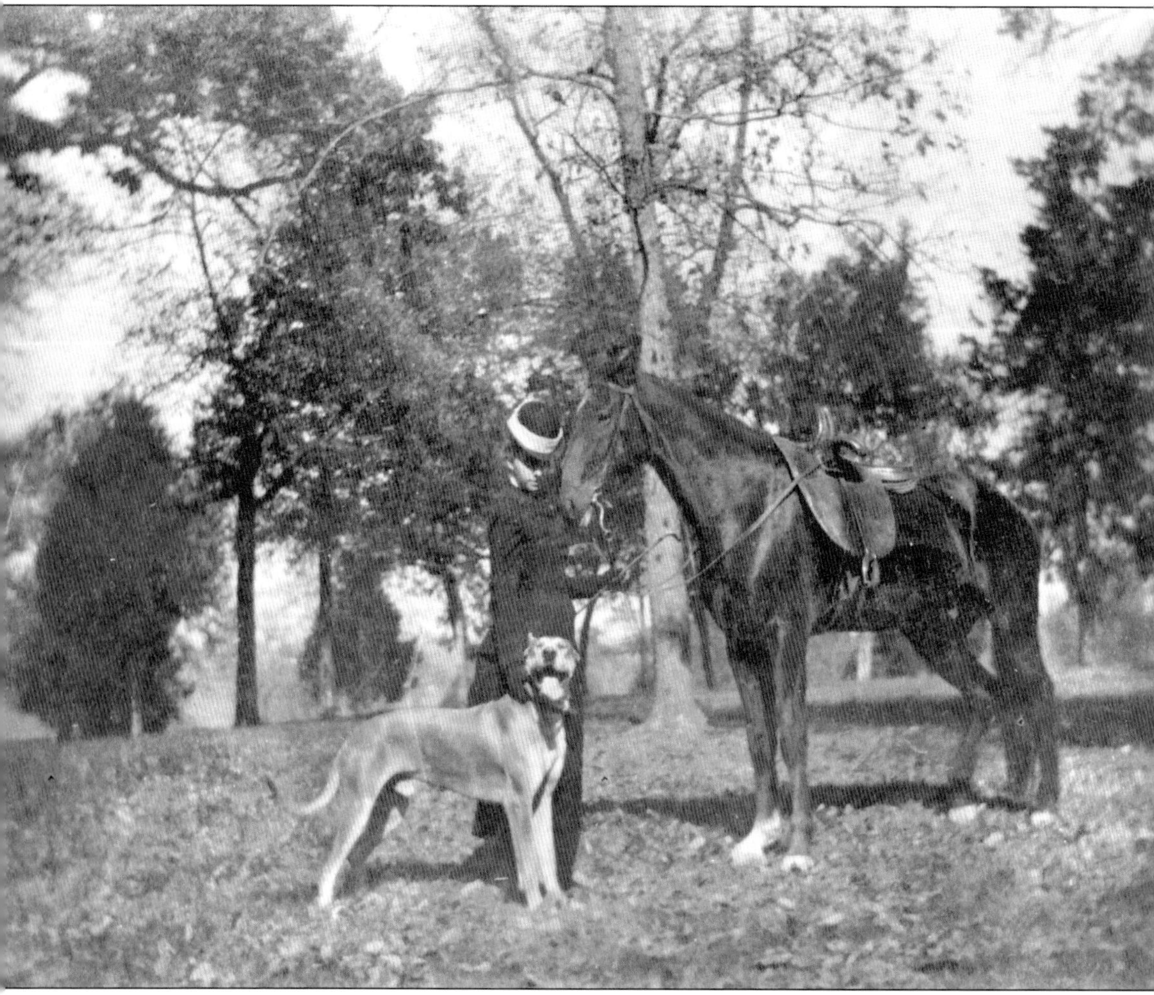

In this *c.* 1900 photograph, an unidentified woman wearing a riding habit stands with a gaited saddle horse and a large dog (possibly a Great Dane) named Rupert. Of particular interest is the woman's sidesaddle. Until the 1920s, it was more acceptable for a woman to ride sidesaddle than to ride astride. The photograph was likely taken at Cloverbottom in Nashville, the site of one of the city's most famous horse racing tracks. (Courtesy of Tennessee State Library and Archives.)

ON THE COVER: The Dickinson children of Travellers Rest in Nashville are pictured here around 1940. They are, from left to right, Rufus, Edith, William, and Maxwell. Their father, Jacob McGavock Dickinson Jr., transformed Travellers Rest into one of the largest Arabian horse farms in the United States. Although they are shown here with their trusted ponies, the children also rode the family's Arabian horses. Dickinson's oldest daughter, Peggy (not pictured), followed in her father's footsteps, breeding Arabians at her Travellers Rest farm in Columbia. (Courtesy of Travellers Rest Plantation and Museum.)

IMAGES
of America

MIDDLE TENNESSEE HORSE BREEDING

Perky Beisel and Rob DeHart

ARCADIA
PUBLISHING

ISBN 978-0-7385-5281-1

Published by Arcadia Publishing
Charleston, South Carolina

Printed in the United States of America

Library of Congress Catalog Card Number: 2007925237

For all general information contact Arcadia Publishing at:
Telephone 843-853-2070
Fax 843-853-0044
E-mail sales@arcadiapublishing.com
For customer service and orders:
Toll-Free 1-888-313-2665

Visit us on the Internet at www.arcadiapublishing.com

To Cooper and Isabelle, the next generation of pony riders

—P. B.

To Clara, Robby, and Goldie

—R. D.

Contents

ACKNOWLEDGMENTS

This book would not have been possible without the help of archival staff at the Tennessee State Library and Archives in Nashville, namely Carol Roberts, Darla Brock, and Karina McDaniel. Photographs credited as TSLA came from the Department of Conservation collection, the library collection, and the Looking Back at Tennessee collection. Dr. Lisa Pruitt of the Albert Gore Sr. Research Center at Middle Tennessee State University in Murfreesboro provided access to the continually exciting Margaret Lindsley Warden Collection. Photographs credited as Gore Center came from the Warden Collection. Some very important contributions were also made by Meyers Brown of the Tennessee State Museum and by Ruth Warner and April McCauley. Special thanks to Peggy Dickinson Fleming; without her generous donation of photographs and documents related to Arabian horse breeding at Travellers Rest, this project may never have gotten off the ground. We would also like to acknowledge the expertise and contributions of Margaret Lindsley Warden and Ridley Wills II to the history of the horse, especially the Thoroughbred, in Middle Tennessee.

INTRODUCTION

Kentucky horse breeder Lewis Sanders lamented in 1836 that "the prevailing opinion in the South is that Tennessee possesses more and better [racehorses] than Kentucky. Tennessee stock will fetch more money in the South than ours will." Indeed, the breeding of fine horses has been both big business and pastime for Middle Tennesseans since settlers first entered the Cumberland Valley in the late 18th century. The fertile pastures and mild climate of the area lent themselves to horse breeding, and the populace embraced the benefits. Horse breeding farms and racetracks were a widespread feature of the pre–Civil War landscape, and practically everyone of means bred horses, whether for sport, transportation, or industry. The extensive involvement of individuals and families in horse sports exemplifies the dedication and resources expended upon horses in Middle Tennessee after 1780. Horse enthusiasts from across the nation traveled to Middle Tennessee to attend its annual breeding farm auctions and compete in its rich races.

It is easy to understand why 19th-century society attached such prestige to breeding horses. For the elite, owning fine horses and demonstrating good horsemanship provided opportunities to establish status. Owning a stallion to stand at stud required a significant capital investment. For instance, in 1835, the cost for a winning three- or four-year-old colt that had yet to prove himself in the breeding shed was $1,000 to $2,000, which would equal about $19,800 to $39,600 in 2007 dollars. Despite the cost, many individuals gambled that the stud fees, which they collected from other horse owners for permission to breed their mares with an accomplished stallion, would more than recover the initial outlay.

Personal and regional disputes were often settled through competitive horse racing. Tennessee's most famous example was the race between future president Andrew Jackson's Truxton and Joseph Erwin's Ploughboy in Nashville in 1806. Jackson had purchased Truxton for $1,500 on May 11, 1805, and was ready to prove that the colt was a credit to his famous sire, *Diomed, who had been imported from Britain (the asterisk indicates a horse imported into the United States). A dispute over the payment of a forfeited race in November 1805 extended past the rescheduled race and resulted in the death of Erwin's son-in-law, Charles Dickinson, from a duel with Jackson on May 30, 1806.

For the working classes, horse racing provided an entertaining diversion, but horses also played a crucial role in their economic pursuits, supplying transport for people and goods and powering American agriculture. Horses and their near cousins, American mules, pulled the plows, planters, and reapers that worked the earth, turned the cane presses and threshing machines, and pulled carts laden with crops to the county market. In urban areas, horses pulled the earliest forms of mass transportation as well as fire engines and road equipment. Most families kept a horse for riding to town or visiting neighbors; doctors often kept a fast-paced horse for long-distance or emergency patient calls; and traveling salesmen and preachers rode or drove to their prospective clientele.

Until the early 20th century, one of the most common businesses in any town or city was the livery stable. These businesses provided temporary stabling for visitors' horses, long-term stabling for nearby residents who did not have the space or inclination to have their own stable or carriage house, and rental horses and carriages for individuals and businesses. Some livery stable owners kept a stallion to breed with local mares, while others specialized in training horses.

African Americans also played an important part in the Middle Tennessee horse industry. The elite entrusted their slaves—and, after the Civil War, their paid farmhands—with the care and training of horses. Nearly every prominent breeder had a favored groomsman to care for his horses. Most antebellum stallion owners who regularly advertised for outside mares added $1 to the breeding fee for the groom. Although the majority of African American men working in the horse industry after the Civil War were grooms, by the 1920s and 1930s, some had made the transition to positions as paid or independent trainers and stable owners. For example, Jerry Nixon had a stable at the Nashville Fair Grounds and taught many elite white Nashvillian children to ride. Whether in the racing industry or the show horse arena, African Americans had vital roles that, nevertheless, were usually unrecognized or limited, despite their talent and knowledge.

With such a robust start, why is Tennessee's legacy of horse breeding and racing frequently eclipsed by that of other areas, such as Kentucky? The answer lies in the equine history of the state, which is as remarkable for its setbacks and interruptions as it is for its triumphs. The Civil War, an often cited setback, devastated the horse industry throughout the South. Confederate cavalry men often bragged that their Southern-bred horses were better than the Federal army's counterparts, but by war's end, hardly any Southern stock survived. Because the Federal army occupied Middle Tennessee for much of the Civil War, the Quartermaster Corps' continual need for horses decreased the available pool of quality horses after the war.

But the horse industry in Middle Tennessee managed to maintain an influential, if not always dominant, role in American horse sports. Part of the region's successful reemergence stemmed from its ability to diversify its breeding stock. Thoroughbred racehorses continued to be a major breeding initiative, but other types of horses, such as the Standardbred, also took root. Developed in the early 19th century from a mixture of Thoroughbreds, local horses, and, especially in Middle Tennessee, the foundation sires of what would become the Tennessee Walking Horse, Standardbreds flourished in the state by the latter part of the 19th century. In Middle Tennessee, pacing Standardbreds, horses who trot with their lateral legs moving together, rather than the more usual diagonal pairs (or trotters), were extremely popular. Although many early Standardbreds raced under saddle, most had a driver in a cart, or sulky.

Middle Tennessee breeders also produced light harness horses (in contrast to heavy harness or draft horses, valued for their brute strength rather than speed) that led the nation in setting speed records and winning match races. The pacer Little Brown Jug, whose sire, Gibson's Tom Hal, passed on the fast Hal strain's pacing style, is one example of a Middle Tennessee horse whose speed earned him national recognition during his lifetime. The top pacing race in the nation was named for Little Brown Jug, who set a one-mile record of 2:11.75.

Once again, politics and economics played a role in the decline of the region's horse industry. A financial panic in 1893 led many of the region's horse breeders to financial ruin, and those who remained in the industry died without heirs, literally or figuratively, to carry on their pursuits. Just as breeders and owners began to rejuvenate Thoroughbred racing after the Civil War, several states began to pass new laws against betting. The Tennessee anti-gambling law, passed in 1905, effectively halted the slow rejuvenation of Thoroughbred flat racing and Standardbred harness racing. The law muted the incentive for Tennesseans to update older tracks, build new tracks, and reform jockey clubs and associations.

At the same time, as older breeders and trainers retired from the business, there were no significant individuals stepping into their place to provide Tennessee racing with much-needed financial backing and leadership. Antebellum breeders, like the Harding and Jackson family at Belle Meade Stud outside of Nashville, had already been slowly losing the local market to the Kentucky competition, and the gambling laws finished the process. Belle Meade had experienced a brief resurgence as a leading breeder and racing stable after the Civil War, especially with *Bonnie Scotland, purchased in 1872; Enquirer, purchased in 1879; and the 1875 homebred Bramble, who attracted stud fees of $100 in 1883. From 1868–1886, Belle Meade, like many other area breeders, sold its yearlings locally each May, and eastern buyers traveled to Nashville for the auction. But Belle Meade, Fairview, Kennesaw, and other Tennessee Thoroughbred producers suffered in the 1890s, as the cost to ship young horses to New York auctions became higher than the sale prices. Finally, rapid suburban development reduced the land holdings of the horse breeding estates located on the edges of the state's urban areas.

Once again, Middle Tennessee horse breeders diversified. Some went into exotic breeds like Arabians, while others aimed to improve the quality and action of work horses in rural areas. Early-20th-century regional breeders continued to cross Saddlebreds (a breed that flourished in Kentucky and Missouri as an upper-class plantation horse noted for its flashy gaits) with Narragansett and Canadian Pacers, Morgans, and Thoroughbreds. They began to develop a new type of riding horse known for its speed (especially those with the Hal bloodlines), strength, and endurance, demonstrated in its signature flat-footed walk, running walk, and canter. The involvement of local farmers and small-scale breeders resulted in a predominately working-class, rural-based breed unique to the state: the Tennessee Walking Horse. In 1935, concerned breeders and owners formed the Tennessee Walking Horse Breeders' and Exhibitors' Association to establish pedigrees by registering horses. The Tennessee Walking Horse was already extremely popular for trail riding, and it was becoming equally well received in the show ring. In 1939, Tennessee Walking Horse owners and trainers began to transform the late-summer Shelbyville horse show in Bedford County into the multimillion-dollar celebration of today.

Of no less importance to the region's economy and reputation was its contribution to the development of the American mule, which played an important role in 19th- and 20th-century southern agriculture and in national militaries. The mule is a cross between a male donkey (a jack) and a female horse (a mare). In Tennessee, Kentucky, and Missouri, the largest producers of mules in the United States at the time, mule breeders often used the American Jack, a breed of donkey developed between 1787 and 1893 from the five main European breeds: Andalusian, Maltese, Catalonia, Majorca, and Poitou. The resulting American Jack stood 15 to 16 hands and weighed 1,000 to 2,000 pounds. Because mules are less prone to colic (a common digestive ailment), less susceptible to extreme heat or cold, and stronger than horses of an equal size, well-bred mules became important investments for farmers and revenue sources for breeders. In 1915, B. C. Hunter of Farmington, Tennessee, advertised his black jack General Logan 4914 with a listing of 14 jack offspring that sold for at least $1,000.

Middle Tennessee breeders and farmers who wanted to sell their jacks and mules usually attended a local, regularly scheduled mule sale day. During World War I, Middle Tennessee provided a large share of the almost 300,000 remount animals to the American Expeditionary Forces in France, which was made up of 32,398 officers, enlisted men, and civilians. In Maury County, the county seat of Columbia had been the site of a large mule and livestock sale since 1840, but in 1934, the traditional event became a festival, complete with parades and activities to entertain spectators while farmers purchased thousands of mules. By the late 1930s, Columbia's Mule Day had became a national event.

As the region's population grew and became more prosperous in the mid-20th century, the Cumberland Valley once again became a leader of American horse breeding and recreational activities. City and county fairs throughout the region vied for participants and spectators with rodeos and benefit horse shows. Foxhunting and steeplechasing flourished in the 1930s throughout Middle Tennessee, but especially south of Nashville. The city of Brentwood became a center of horse breeding and sporting activities during the early 1940s. The post–World War II boom supported the growth of youth-oriented activities and associations organized by Nashville horse enthusiast and journalist Margaret Lindsley Warden, including the Interschool Riding Tournament, the Horse Sense one-day trial (sponsored by the *Nashville Tennessean*), and the Middle Tennessee Pony Club.

From the 1970s to 2005, the fifth generation of Middle Tennessean breeders and horse enthusiasts celebrated golden anniversaries while participating in an increasingly varied range of activities, including polo, competitive trail riding, hunting, and jumping.

Today the horse continues to play an important role in Middle Tennessee's economy and society, but many of the historic properties and sites associated with the region's early equine successes have been lost to suburban development. The following seven chapters will provide an introduction to Middle Tennessee's equine history while highlighting a few of the numerous horses, individuals, facilities, and events that comprise the region's heritage of horse breeding and sports.

One

1780–1865

"This, I suppose, is the acknowledged center of the race horse region," wrote William Giles Harding to *The American Turf Register* from his Belle Meade horse farm in Davidson County in 1839. "Blood stock here is all the go. To be without it is to be out of fashion and destitute of taste. So I, too, have procured a little of the real grit which by and by I hope to increase." Forty years earlier, horse breeders in Sumner County—and Gallatin in particular—had introduced Tennessee to Thoroughbred racehorses from Virginia. It was not long before elites throughout the region recognized the financial and social rewards of breeding prizewinning horses. Horses bred in Middle Tennessee before the Civil War raced successfully throughout the South.

Traveling through Middle Tennessee today reveals little of the region's former obsession with horse racing. The numerous racetracks that filled the landscape, at one time the pride of each ambitious county and city, have long been covered over. Only a handful of historic sites survive to tell the stories of the famous horses and breeders who lived in the region. While this history is obscured, it is not lost. Documentary evidence in the form of newspapers, broadsides, portraits, and a few rare photographs recall Middle Tennessee's history of horse breeding before the conclusion of the American Civil War.

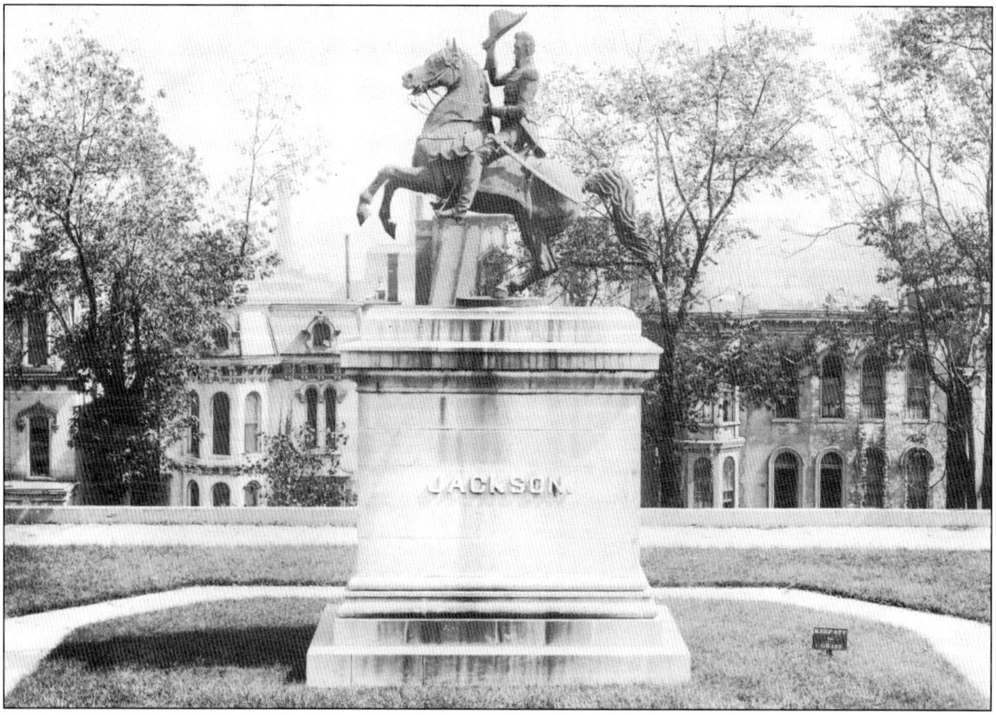

Representing Tennessee's most famous horseman, this Clark Mills bronze statue of Gen. Andrew Jackson at the Battle of New Orleans rests on the lawn of the Tennessee State Capitol in Nashville. Although Jackson had sold most of his Thoroughbred breeding stock by 1816, he continued to own and race horses while serving as president of the United States. (Courtesy of TSLA.)

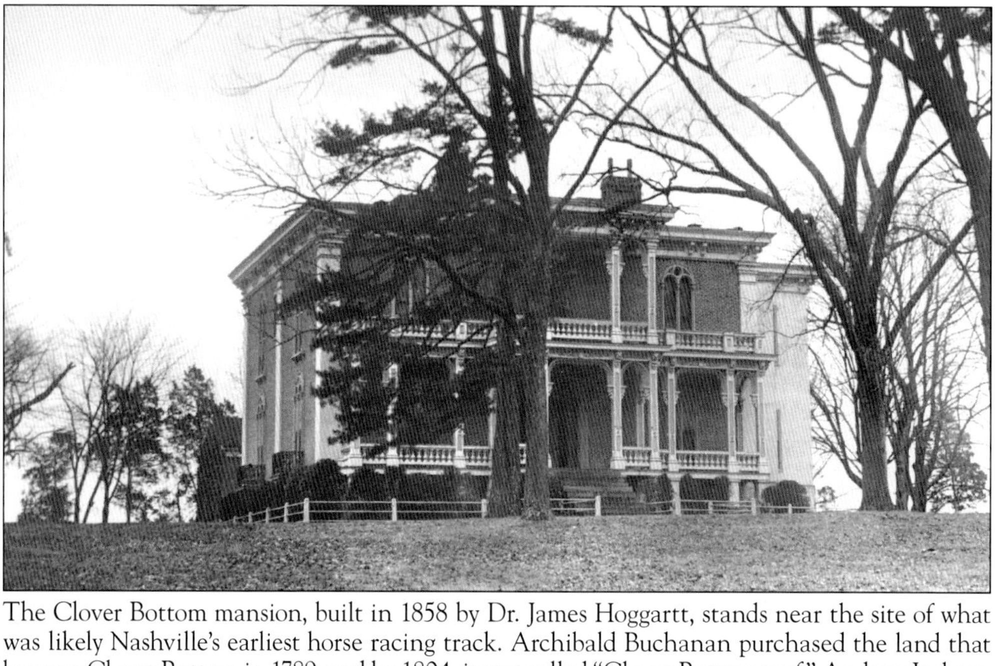

The Clover Bottom mansion, built in 1858 by Dr. James Hoggartt, stands near the site of what was likely Nashville's earliest horse racing track. Archibald Buchanan purchased the land that became Clover Bottom in 1789, and by 1804, it was called "Clover Bottom turf." Andrew Jackson purchased an interest in the track the following year. (Courtesy of TSLA.)

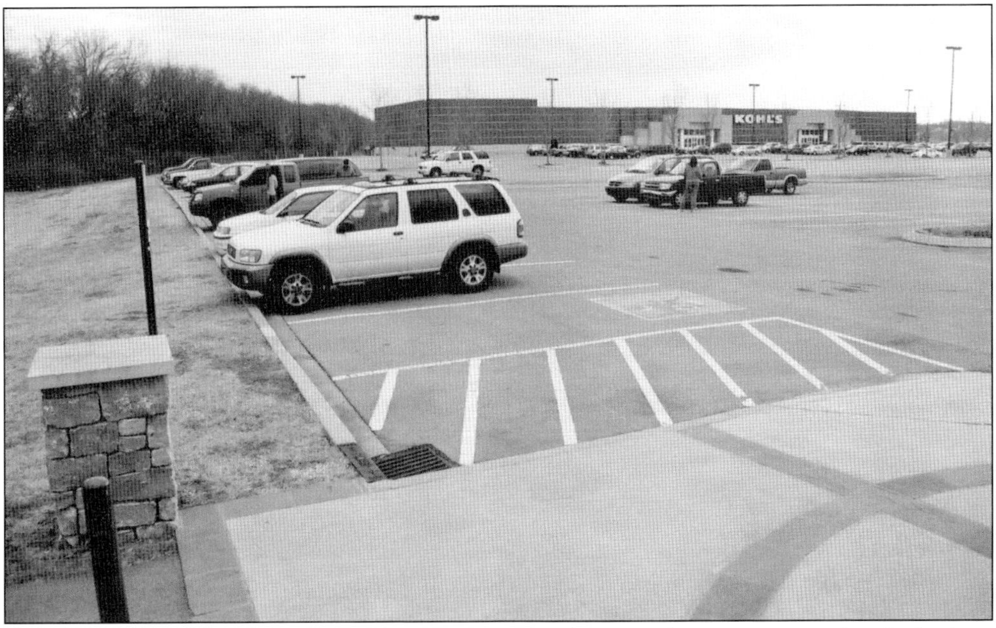

These two photographs depict contemporary views of racetrack sites associated with Andrew Jackson: Clover Bottom (above) and Gallatin Track (below). Today a Kohl's department store is near the area of the once-infamous Clover Bottom track. It was here that, in 1806, Jackson's Truxton raced Joseph Erwin's Ploughboy. Truxton was the victor, despite being lame in two legs and having a sprung shoe on a third leg. A year-long dispute over the race led to a duel between Jackson and Erwin's son-in-law Charles Dickinson, resulting in Dickinson's death. Since the early 20th century, a railroad depot has sat in place of the Gallatin Track's grandstands in Sumner County. The Gallatin Track was the site of the state's first official horse race in 1804. Jackson's Indian Queen was defeated by Sumner County breeder Dr. Redmond Barry's Polly Medley. (Photographs by April McCauley.)

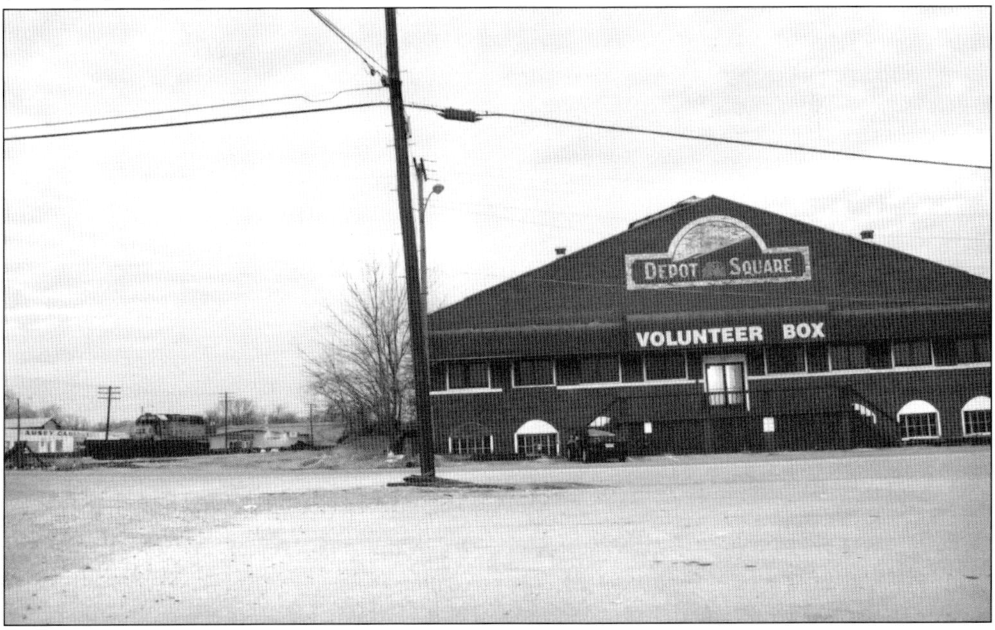

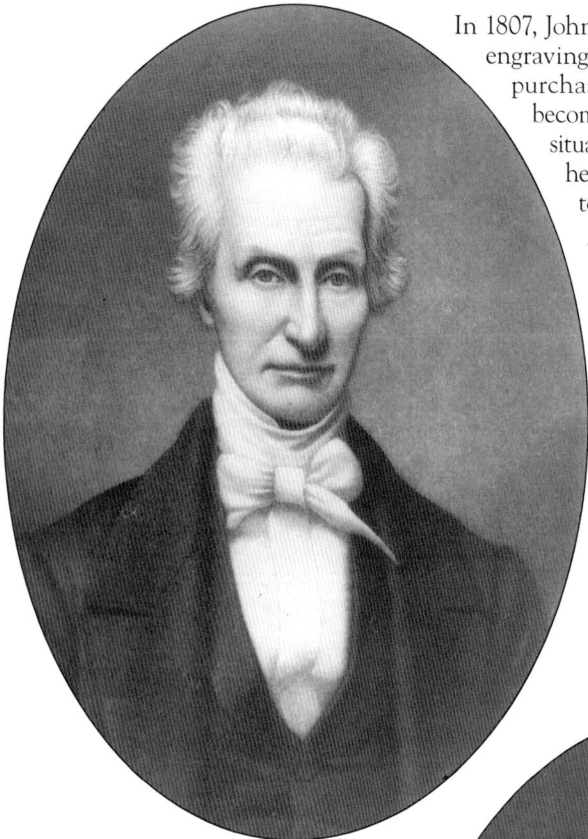

In 1807, John Harding (1777–1865), depicted in this engraving from a Washington B. Cooper portrait, purchased the first 250 acres of what would become the 5,300-acre Belle Meade Plantation, situated seven miles south of Nashville. Before he turned management of Belle Meade over to his son William Giles Harding in 1839, John Harding established Thoroughbred horse breeding at the site. (Courtesy of Gore Center.)

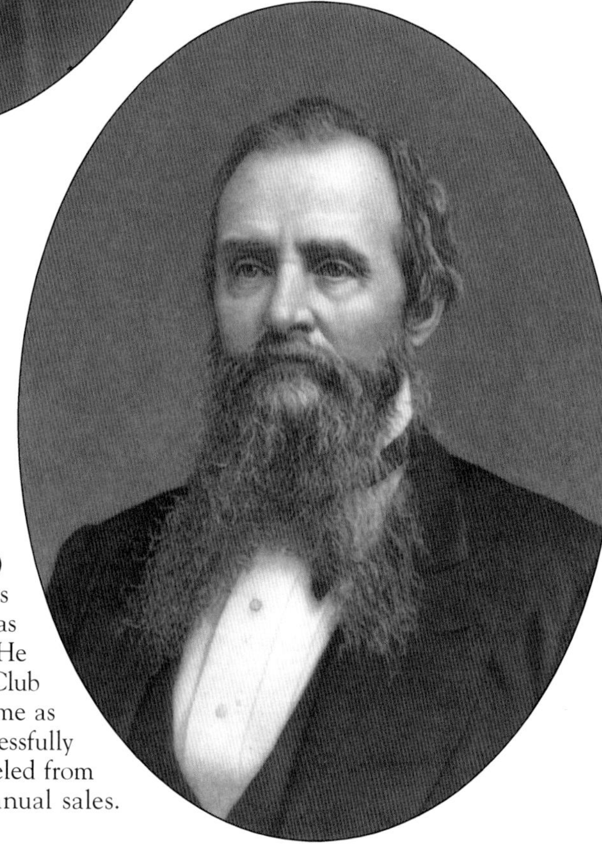

William Giles Harding (1808–1886) continued his father's horse pursuits and began Belle Meade's reputation as a leading Thoroughbred horse farm. He presided over the Nashville Jockey Club in 1856, and he gained national fame as a producer of horses that raced successfully throughout the South. Buyers traveled from across the nation to the stud's annual sales. (Courtesy of TSLA.)

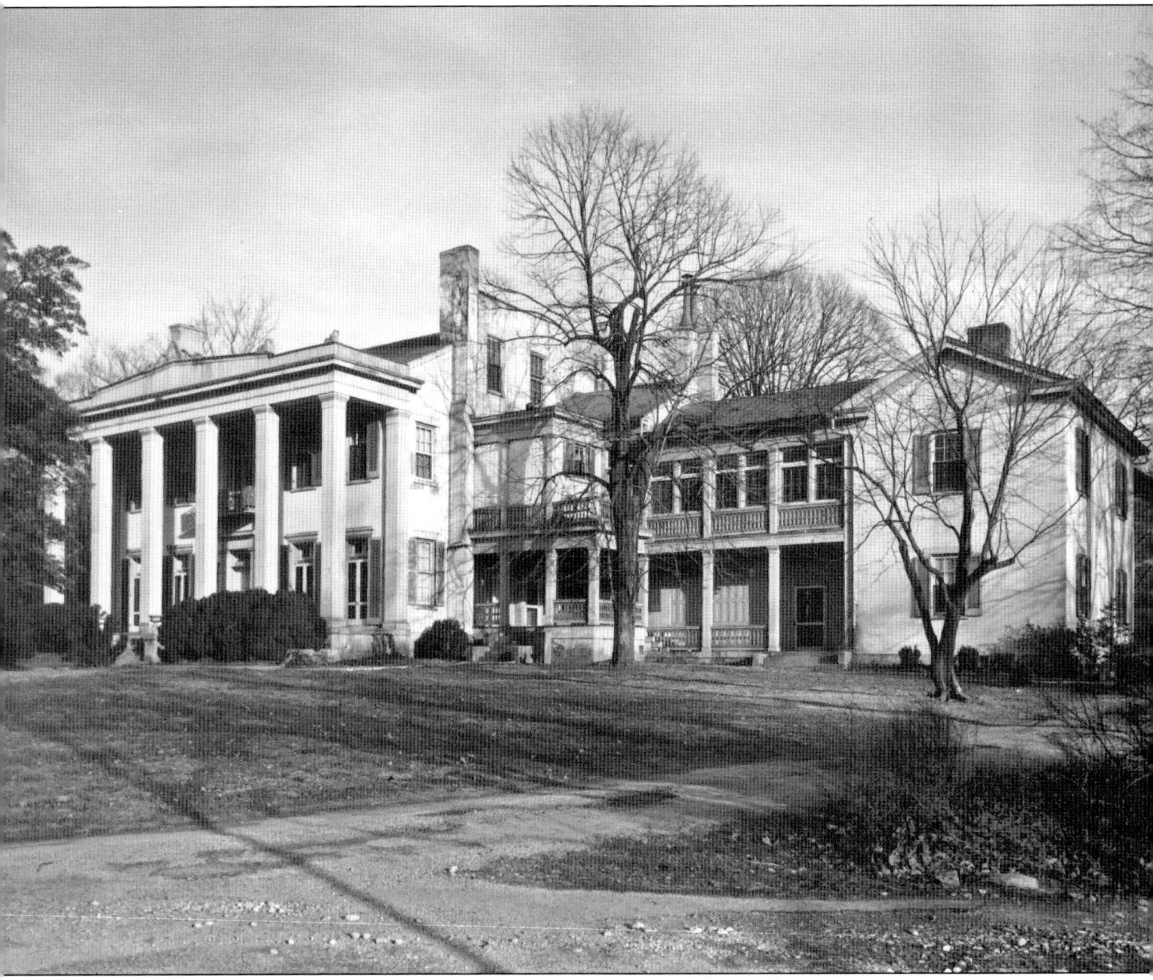

From 1853 to 1854, William Giles Harding oversaw a Greek Revival reconstruction of his father's 1820 Federal-style house. This is the Belle Meade Mansion that visitors see today when they tour the historic site, which is owned by the Association for the Preservation of Tennessee Antiquities. The Hardings bred horses in Nashville at a time when the state of Tennessee had at least 10 established racetracks and over 20 organized jockey clubs. As happened throughout most of the South, the Civil War devastated the Hardings' horse breeding stock. In 1862, William's wife, Elizabeth, complained to the federally appointed military governor of the state, Andrew Johnson, that the federal government "has made a requisition upon me for horses for the use of the cavalry and have taken every suitable horse I had except my carriage horses." Nonetheless, Belle Meade managed to survive the Federal army's occupation of Nashville and reemerge as a world-renowned breeder of Thoroughbreds following the war. (Courtesy of TSLA.)

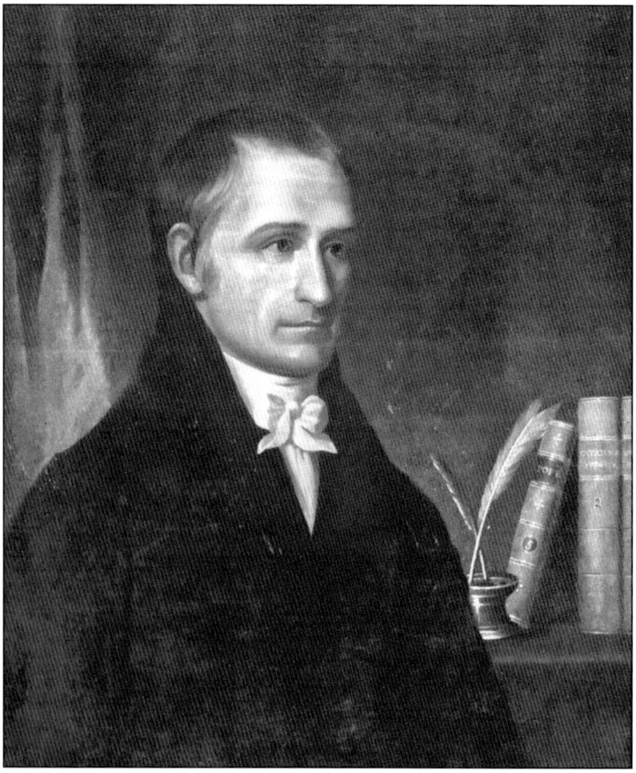

This Ralph E. W. Earl portrait depicts Judge John Overton (1766–1833) of Travellers Rest in Nashville. He did not breed horses on the scale of men such as Andrew Jackson and the Hardings, but, like many Middle Tennessee elites, he invested in fine horses in order to collect stud fees. In the 1830 letter seen at right, one of his agents advised him not to send the stallion *Bagdad to West Tennessee to stud because of the large number of quality stallions already in the area for the season. *Bagdad was an Arabian horse bred in Syria and imported into the United States in 1822. Well-regarded stallions often had a large number of investors, who earned or lost money depending on the success of the stallion's offspring. (Above courtesy of Travellers Rest Plantation and Museum; at right courtesy of TSLA.)

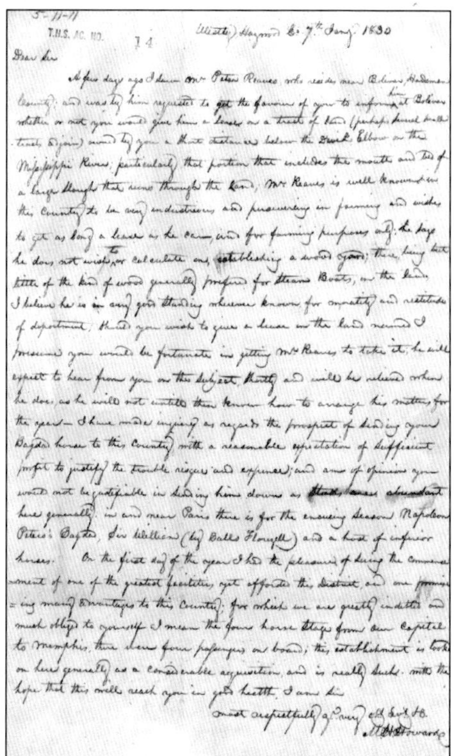

5-11-11
T.H.S. AC. NO. 14
[illegible] Haywood Co. 7th Jany. 1830

Dear Sir

A few days ago I saw Mr Peter Reaves, who resides near Bolivar, Hardeman County; and was by him requested to ask the favour of you to inform him at Bolivar whether or not you would give him a lease on a tract of land (perhaps several [illegible] tracts adjoin) owned by you a short distance below the Devil's Elbow on the Mississippi River, particularly that portion that includes the mouth and [illegible] of a large slough that runs through the land, Mr Reaves is well known in this County to be very industrious and persevering in farming and wishes to get as long a lease as he can, and for farming purposes only; he says he does not wish to or calculate on establishing a wood yard; there being but little of the kind of wood generally prefered for Steam Boats, on the land. I believe he is in very good standing wherever known for [illegible] and rectitude of deportment, should you wish to give a lease on the land named I presume you would be fortunate in getting Mr Reaves to take it, he will expect to hear from you on this subject shortly and will be relieved when he does, as he will not untill then know how to arrange his matters for the year— I have made inquiry as regards the prospect of sending your Bagdad horse to this County with a reasonable expectation of sufficient profit to justify the trouble risque and expence; and am of opinion you would not be justifiable in sending him down as ~~[illegible]~~ abundant here generally. in and near Paris there is for the ensuing season Napoleon Peters' Bagdad, Sir William (by Balls Florizell) and a host of inferior horses. On the first day of the year I had the pleasure of seeing the commencement of one of the greatest facilities yet afforded this District, and one promising many advantages to this Country; for which we are greatly indebted and much obliged to yourself I mean the four horse Stage from our Capital to Memphis, there were four passengers on board; this establishment is looked on here generally as a considerable acquisition, and is really such. with the hope that this will reach you in good health, I am Sir

most respectfully yr very obt Servt &c.
[illegible] Howard

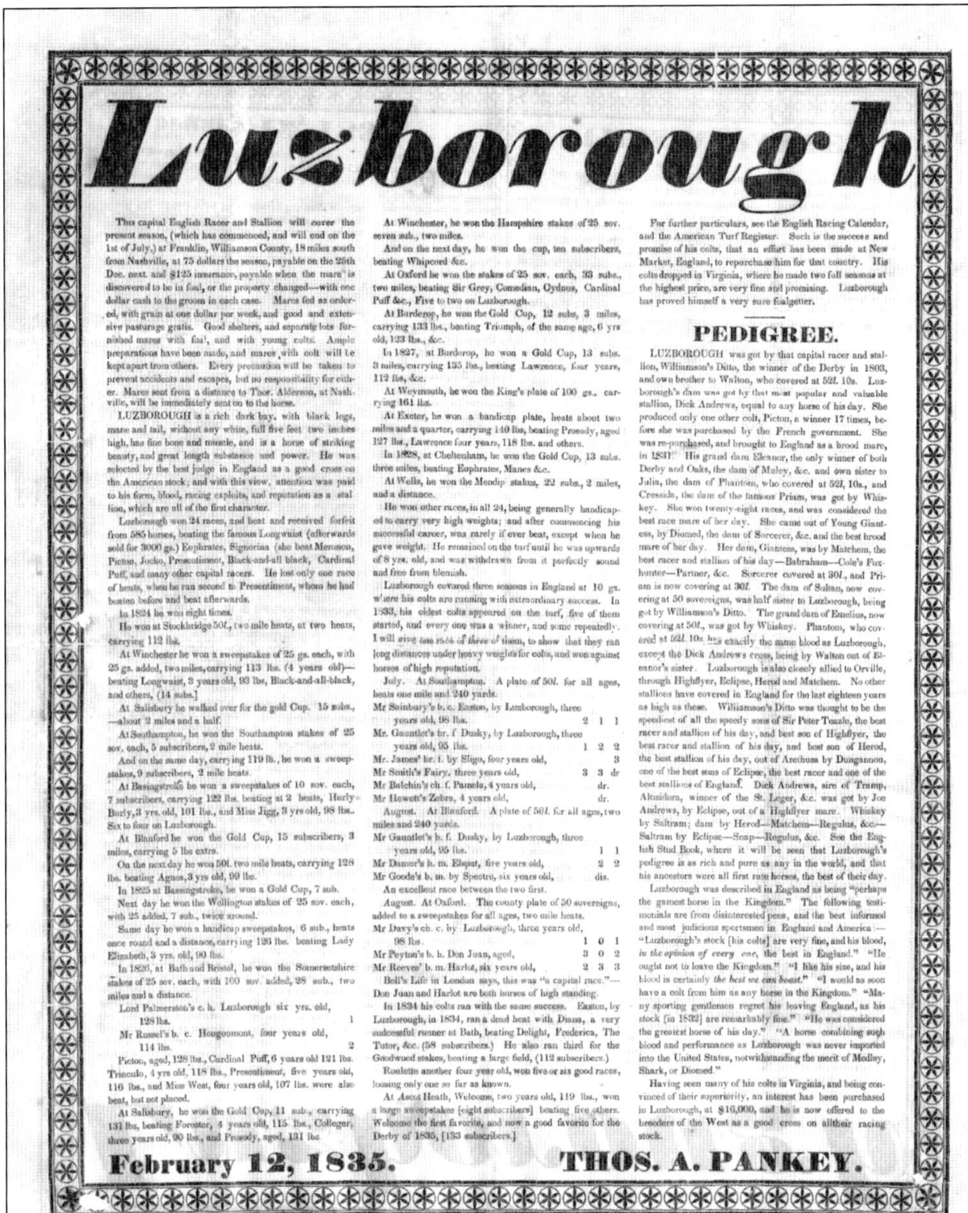

Luzborough

This capital English Racer and Stallion will cover the present season, (which has commenced, and will end on the 1st of July,) at Franklin, Williamson County, 18 miles south from Nashville, at 75 dollars the season, payable on the 25th Dec. next. and $125 insurance, payable when the mare is discovered to be in foal, or the property changed—with one dollar cash to the groom in each case. Mares fed as ordered, with grain at one dollar per week, and good and extensive pasturage gratis. Good shelters, and separate lots furnished mares with foal, and with young colts. Ample preparations have been made, and mares with colt will be kept apart from others. Every precaution will be taken to prevent accidents and escapes, but no responsibility for either. Mares sent from a distance to Thos. Alderson, at Nashville, will be immediately sent on to the horse.

LUZBOROUGH is a rich dark bay, with black legs, mane and tail, without any white, full five feet two inches high, has fine bone and muscle, and is a horse of striking beauty, and great length substance and power. He was selected by the best judge in England as a good cross on the American stock; and with this view, attention was paid to his form, blood, racing exploits, and reputation as a stallion, which are all of the first character.

Luzborough won 24 races, and beat and received forfeit from 585 horses, beating the famous Longwaist (afterwards sold for 3000 gs.) Euphrates, Signorina (she beat Memnon, Picton, Jocko, Presentiment, Black-and-all black, Cardinal Puff, and many other capital racers. He lost only one race of heats, when he ran second to Presentiment, whom he had beaten before and beat afterwards.

In 1824 he won eight times.

He won at Stockbridge 50*l*., two mile heats, at two heats, carrying 112 lbs.

At Winchester he won a sweepstakes of 25 gs. each, with 25 gs. added, two miles, carrying 113 lbs. (4 years old)—beating Longwaist, 3 years old, 93 lbs, Black-and-all-black, and others, (14 subs.]

At Salisbury he walked over for the gold Cup. 15 subs., —about 2 miles and a half.

At Southampton, he won the Southampton stakes of 25 sov. each, 5 subscribers, 2 mile heats.

And on the same day, carrying 119 lb., he won a sweepstakes, 9 subscribers, 2 mile heats.

At Basingstroke he won a sweepstakes of 10 sov. each, 7 subscribers, carrying 122 lbs. beating at 2 heats, Hurly-Burly, 3 yrs. old, 101 lbs., and Miss Jigg, 3 yrs old, 98 lbs.. Six to four on Luzborough.

At Blanford he won the Gold Cup, 15 subscribers, 3 miles, carrying 5 lbs extra.

On the next day he won 50l. two mile heats, carrying 128 lbs. beating Agnes, 3 yrs old, 99 lbs.

In 1825 at Bassingstroke, he won a Gold Cup, 7 sub.

Next day he won the Wellington stakes of 25 sov. each, with 25 added, 7 sub., twice around.

Same day he won a handicap sweepstakes, 6 sub., heats once round and a distance, carrying 126 lbs. beating Lady Elizabeth, 3 yrs. old, 90 lbs.

In 1826, at Bath and Bristol, he won the Somersetshire stakes of 25 sov. each, with 100 sov. added, 28 sub., two miles and a distance.

Lord Palmerston's c. h. Luzborough six yrs. old, 128 lbs. 1
Mr Russel's b. c. Hougoumont, four years old, 114 lbs. 2

Picton, aged, 128 lbs., Cardinal Puff, 6 years old 121 lbs. Trinculo, 4 yrs old, 118 lbs., Presentiment, five years old, 116 lbs., and Miss West, four years old, 107 lbs. were also beat, but not placed.

At Salisbury, he won the Gold Cup, 11 sub., carrying 131 lbs, beating Forester, 4 years old, 115 lbs., Colleger, three years old, 90 lbs., and Prosody, aged, 131 lbs.

At Winchester, he won the Hampshire stakes of 25 sov. seven sub., two miles.

And on the next day, he won the cup, ten subscribers, beating Whipcord &c.

At Oxford he won the stakes of 25 sov. each, 33 subs., two miles, beating Sir Grey, Comedian, Cydnus, Cardinal Puff &c., Five to two on Luzborough.

At Burderop, he won the Gold Cup, 12 subs, 3 miles, carrying 133 lbs., beating Triumph, of the same age, 6 yrs old, 123 lbs., &c.

In 1827, at Burderop, he won a Gold Cup, 13 subs. 3 miles, carrying 135 lbs., beating Lawrence, four years, 112 lbs, &c.

At Weymouth, he won the King's plate of 100 gs., carrying 161 lbs.

At Exeter, he won a handicap plate, heats about two miles and a quarter, carrying 140 lbs, beating Prosody, aged 127 lbs., Lawrence four years, 118 lbs. and others.

In 1828, at Cheltenham, he won the Gold Cup, 13 subs. three miles, beating Euphrates, Manes &c.

At Wells, he won the Mendip stakes, 22 subs., 2 miles, and a distance.

He won other races, in all 24, being generally handicapped to carry very high weights; and after commencing his successful career, was rarely if ever beat, except when he gave weight. He remained on the turf until he was upwards of 8 yrs. old, and was withdrawn from it perfectly sound and free from blemish.

Luzborough covered three seasons in England at 10 gs. where his colts are running with extraordinary success. In 1833, his oldest colts appeared on the turf, five of them started, and every one was a winner, and some repeatedly. I will give one race of three of them, to show that they ran long distances under heavy weights for colts, and won against horses of high reputation.

July. At Southampton. A plate of 50*l*. for all ages, heats one mile and 240 yards.

Mr Sainbury's b. c. Easton, by Luzborough, three years old, 98 lbs. 2 1 1
Mr. Gauntlet's br. f Dusky, by Luzborough, three years old, 95 lbs. 1 2 2
Mr. James' br. f. by Sligo, four years old, 3
Mr Smith's Fairy, three years old, 3 3 dr
Mr Balchin's ch. f. Pamela, 4 years old, dr.
Mr Hewett's Zebra, 4 years old, dr.

August. At Blanford. A plate of 50*l*. for all ages, two miles and 240 yards.

Mr Gauntlet's b. f. Dusky, by Luzborough, three years old, 95 lbs. 1 1
Mr Damer's b. m. Elspat, five years old, 2 2
Mr Goode's b. m. by Spectre, six years old, dis.

An excellent race between the two first.

August. At Oxford. The county plate of 50 sovereigns, added to a sweepstakes for all ages, two mile heats.

Mr Davy's ch. c. by Luzborough, three years old, 98 lbs. 1 0 1
Mr Peyton's b. h. Don Juan, aged, 3 0 2
Mr Reeves' b. m. Harlot, six years old, 2 3 3

Bell's Life in London says, this was "a capital race."—Don Juan and Harlot are both horses of high standing.

In 1834 his colts ran with the same success. Easton, by Luzborough, in 1834, ran a dead heat with Diana, a very successful runner at Bath, beating Delight, Frederica, The Tutor, &c. (58 subscribers.) He also ran third for the Goodwood stakes, beating a large field, (112 subscribers.)

Roulette another four year old, won five or six good races, loosing only one so far as known.

At Ascot Heath, Welcome, two years old, 119 lbs., won a large sweepstakes [eight subscribers] beating five others. Welcome the first favorite, and now a good favorite for the Derby of 1835, [133 subscribers.]

For further particulars, see the English Racing Calendar, and the American Turf Register. Such is the success and promise of his colts, that an effort has been made at New Market, England, to repurchase him for that country. His colts dropped in Virginia, where he made two full seasons at the highest price, are very fine and promising. Luzborough has proved himself a very sure foalgetter.

PEDIGREE.

LUZBOROUGH was got by that capital racer and stallion, Williamson's Ditto, the winner of the Derby in 1803, and own brother to Walton, who covered at 52*l*. 10s. Luzborough's dam was got by that most popular and valuable stallion, Dick Andrews, equal to any horse of his day. She produced only one other colt, Picton, a winner 17 times, before she was purchased by the French government. She was re-purchased, and brought to England as a brood mare, in 1831. His grand dam Eleanor, the only winner of both Derby and Oaks, the dam of Muley, &c. and own sister to Julia, the dam of Phantom, who covered at 52*l*, 10s., and Cresside, the dam of the famous Priam, was got by Whiskey. She won twenty-eight races, and was considered the best race mare of her day. She came out of Young Giantess, by Diomed, the dam of Sorcerer, &c. and the best brood mare of her day. Her dam, Giantess, was by Matchem, the best racer and stallion of his day—Babraham—Cole's Foxhunter—Partner, &c. Sorcerer covered at 30*l*., and Priam is now covering at 30*l*. The dam of Sultan, now covering at 50 sovereigns, was half sister to Luzborough, being got by Williamson's Ditto. The grand dam of Emelius, now covering at 50*l*., was got by Whiskey. Phantom, who covered at 52*l*. 10s. has exactly the same blood as Luzborough, except the Dick Andrews cross, being by Walton out of Eleanor's sister. Luzborough is also closely allied to Orville, through Highflyer, Eclipse, Herod and Matchem. No other stallions have covered in England for the last eighteen years as high as these. Williamson's Ditto was thought to be the speediest of all the speedy sons of Sir Peter Teazle, the best racer and stallion of his day, and best son of Highflyer, the best racer and stallion of his day, and best son of Herod, the best stallion of his day, out of Arethusa by Dungannon, one of the best sons of Eclipse, the best racer and one of the best stallions of England. Dick Andrews, sire of Tramp, Altisidora, winner of the St. Leger, &c. was got by Joe Andrews, by Eclipse, out of a Highflyer mare. Whiskey by Saltram; dam by Herod—Matchem—Regulus, &c.—Saltram by Eclipse—Snap—Regulus, &c. See the English Stud Book, where it will be seen that Luzborough's pedigree is as rich and pure as any in the world, and that his ancestors were all first rate horses, the best of their day.

Luzborough was described in England as being "perhaps the gamest horse in the Kingdom." The following testimonials are from disinterested pens, and the best informed and most judicious sportsmen in England and America:—"Luzborough's stock [his colts] are very fine, and his blood, *in the opinion of every one*, the best in England." "He ought not to leave the Kingdom." "I like his size, and his blood is certainly *the best we can boast*." "I would as soon have a colt from him as any horse in the Kingdom." "Many sporting gentlemen regret his leaving England, as his stock [in 1832] are remarkably fine." "He was considered the greatest horse of his day." "A horse combining such blood and performance as Luzborough was never imported into the United States, notwithstanding the merit of Medley, Shark, or Diomed."

Having seen many of his colts in Virginia, and being convinced of their superiority, an interest has been purchased in Luzborough, at $16,000, and he is now offered to the breeders of the West as a good cross on alltheir racing stock.

February 12, 1835. **THOS. A. PANKEY.**

S. Nye & Co. Printers..Republican Office, Nashville.

This 1835 broadside advertises the availability of the famed Thoroughbred stallion *Luzborough to stud in Williamson County. *Luzborough was foaled (born) in England in 1820 and was later imported into the United States. In the 1835 season, a horse owner would have to pay $75 for the chance to mate a mare with *Luzborough. In just two years, *Luzborough's stockholders collected a reported $20,000 in stud fees. With so much money changing hands, it is not surprising that fierce rivalries developed between investors of competing horses. The owners of *Luzborough and those of his nearest rival, *Leviathan, frequently challenged each other in the press to test the qualities of these stallions' bloodlines through races that featured their offspring. These rivalries sometimes expanded, pitting breeders of one state against those of another state and sparking regional competitions between the North and South. (Courtesy of TSLA.)

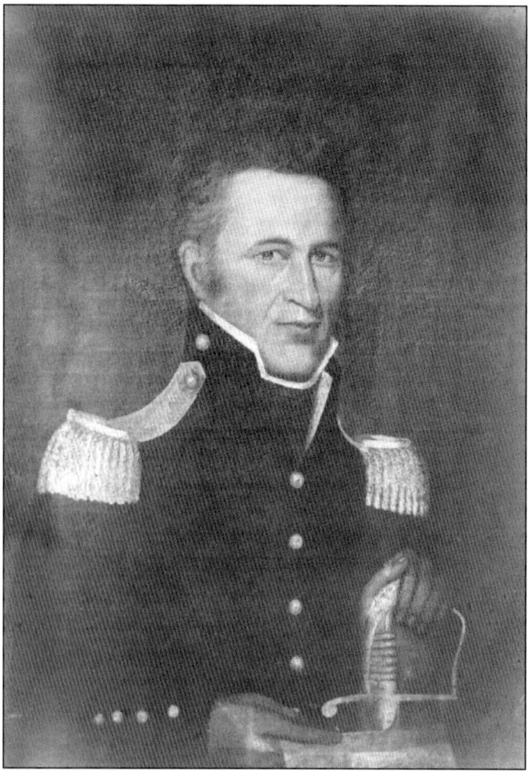

Col. George Elliott was one of a number of prominent Thoroughbred horse breeders is Sumner County. His mare Black Sophia gained fame when she won a race against descendants of Andrew Jackson's Truxton in 1820. Elliott's farm, Wall Spring, also stabled the important stallion *Leviathan, along with several other stallions, making the stud an important site in Middle Tennessee antebellum Thoroughbred breeding. (Courtesy of TSLA.)

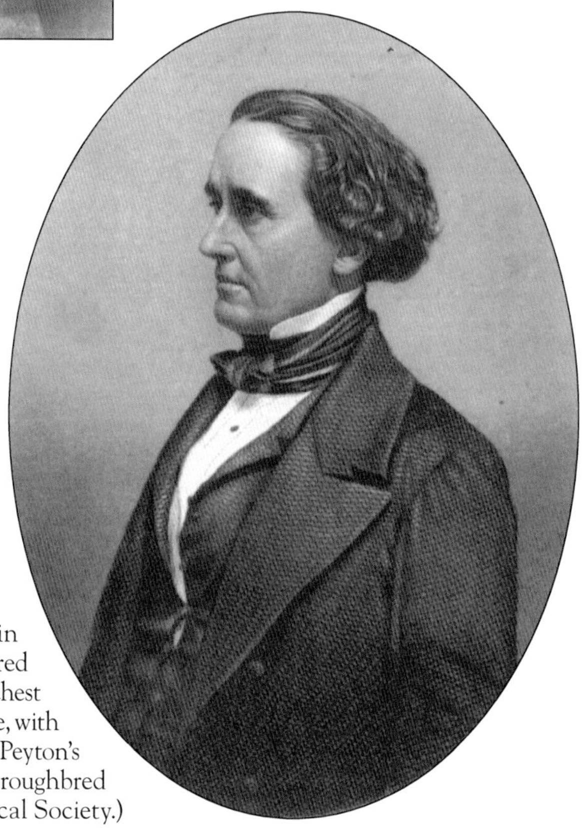

As well as representing Sumner County in the U.S. Congress, Balie Peyton sponsored the 1843 Peyton Stakes in Nashville, the richest horse race run in the country up to that time, with a purse of $35,000. Prior to the Civil War, Peyton's farm Station Camp was a renowned Thoroughbred nursery. (Courtesy of Tennessee Historical Society.)

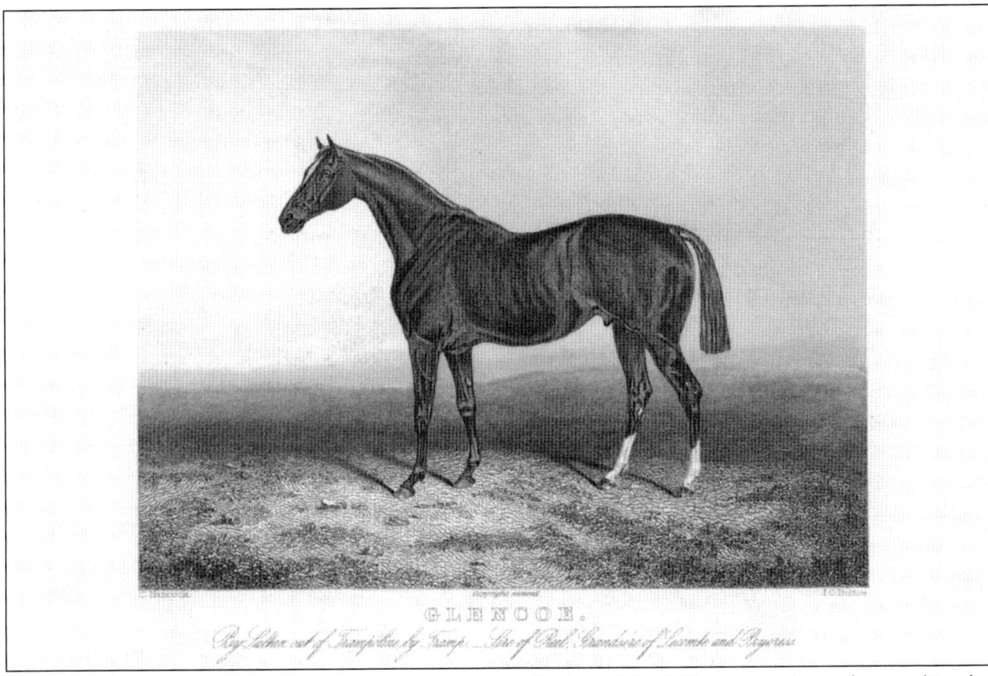

Peytona, the winner of the Peyton Stakes, was sired (fathered) by *Glencoe, who is depicted in this engraving of a painting by Edward Troye. *Glencoe was one of the most successful Thoroughbred stallions to stand in the South. A New York investor imported him from England. Between 1840 and 1848, *Glencoe produced an estimated 481 foals while standing in Tennessee, Alabama, and Kentucky. (Courtesy of Gore Center.)

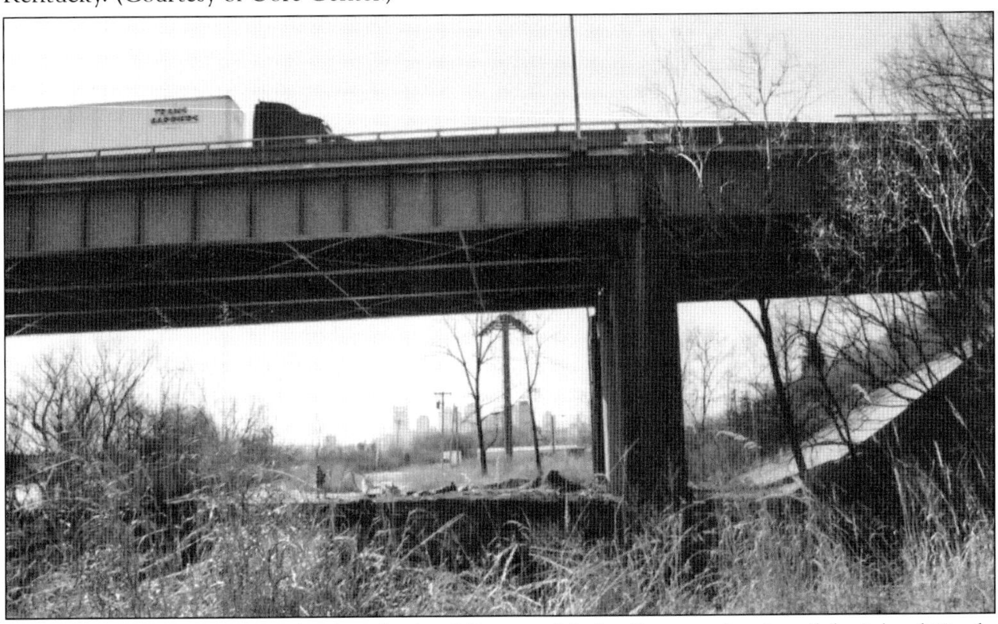

Today Interstate 65 crosses the Cumberland River in Nashville near the site of the Island Track, which hosted the Peyton Stakes. Also called the Nashville Track or Burns Island Track, it opened as one of the city's premier horse racing tracks in 1828. Periodic flooding forced the track's closure by 1887. (Photograph by April McCauley.)

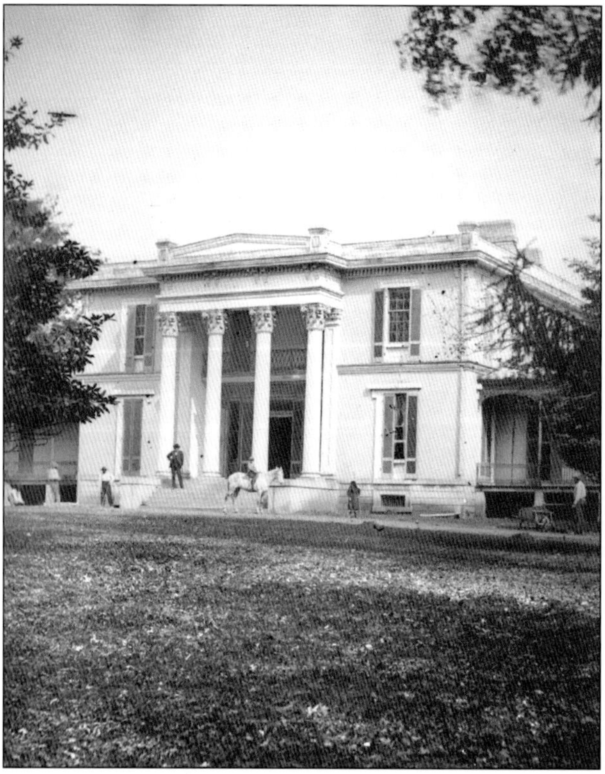

Ashwood Hall in Maury County, seen in this late-19th-century photograph, was the antebellum home of Leonidas Polk (1806–1864). The members of the Polk family were avid racehorse breeders. Although men like Leonidas Polk laid the foundation for horse breeding in Maury County, the region did not emerge as a leader in the field until after the Civil War. (Courtesy of TSLA.)

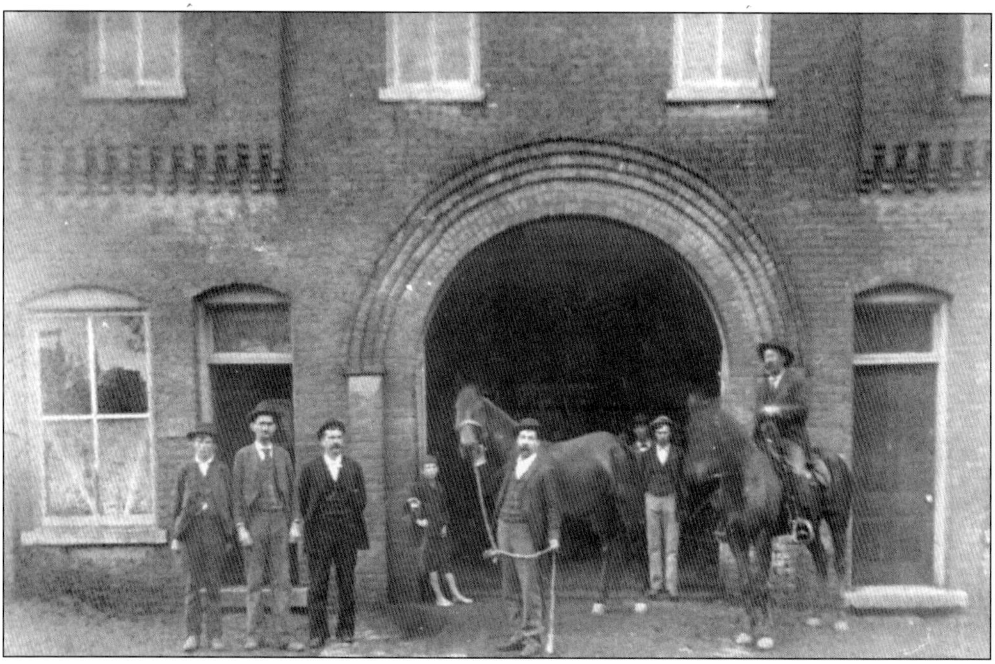

This *c.* 1896 photograph shows the G. W. Davis Saloon and Livery in Lewisburg. Liveries were common in towns and cities both before and after the Civil War. They provided both temporary and long-term stabling for horses, as well as rental horses and carriages. Most livery stables were near the downtown business district. (Courtesy of TSLA.)

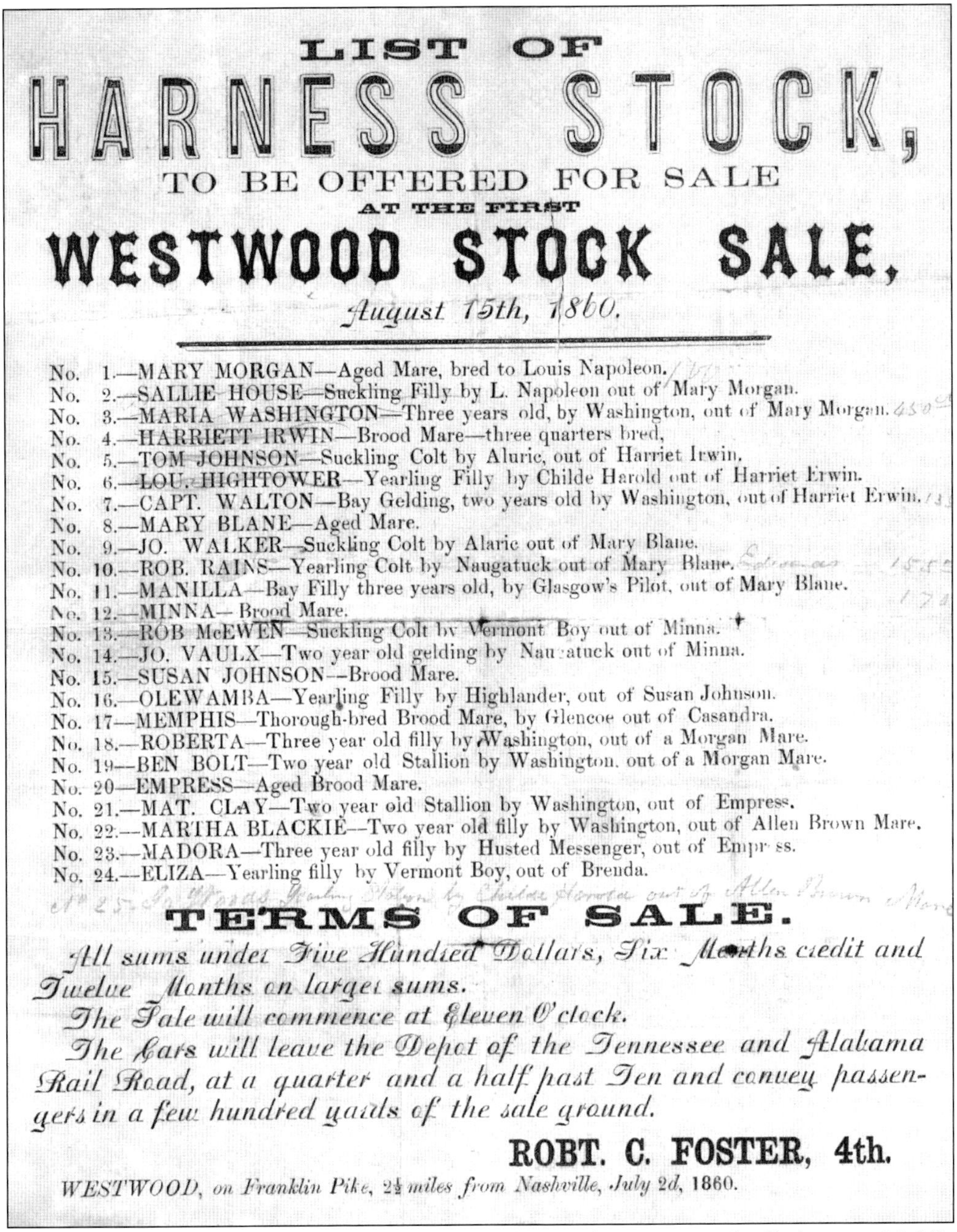

LIST OF

HARNESS STOCK,

TO BE OFFERED FOR SALE

AT THE FIRST

WESTWOOD STOCK SALE,

August 15th, 1860.

No. 1.—MARY MORGAN—Aged Mare, bred to Louis Napoleon.
No. 2.—SALLIE HOUSE—Suckling Filly by L. Napoleon out of Mary Morgan.
No. 3.—MARIA WASHINGTON—Three years old, by Washington, out of Mary Morgan.
No. 4.—HARRIETT IRWIN—Brood Mare—three quarters bred,
No. 5.—TOM JOHNSON—Suckling Colt by Aluric, out of Harriet Irwin.
No. 6.—LOU. HIGHTOWER—Yearling Filly by Childe Harold out of Harriet Erwin.
No. 7.—CAPT. WALTON—Bay Gelding, two years old by Washington, out of Harriet Erwin.
No. 8.—MARY BLANE—Aged Mare.
No. 9.—JO. WALKER—Suckling Colt by Alaric out of Mary Blane.
No. 10.—ROB. RAINS—Yearling Colt by Naugatuck out of Mary Blane.
No. 11.—MANILLA—Bay Filly three years old, by Glasgow's Pilot, out of Mary Blane.
No. 12.—MINNA—Brood Mare.
No. 13.—ROB McEWEN—Suckling Colt by Vermont Boy out of Minna.
No. 14.—JO. VAULX—Two year old gelding by Naugatuck out of Minna.
No. 15.—SUSAN JOHNSON—Brood Mare.
No. 16.—OLEWAMBA—Yearling Filly by Highlander, out of Susan Johnson.
No. 17—MEMPHIS—Thorough-bred Brood Mare, by Glencoe out of Casandra.
No. 18.—ROBERTA—Three year old filly by Washington, out of a Morgan Mare.
No. 19—BEN BOLT—Two year old Stallion by Washington, out of a Morgan Mare.
No. 20—EMPRESS—Aged Brood Mare.
No. 21.—MAT. CLAY—Two year old Stallion by Washington, out of Empress.
No. 22.—MARTHA BLACKIE—Two year old filly by Washington, out of Allen Brown Mare.
No. 23.—MADORA—Three year old filly by Husted Messenger, out of Empress.
No. 24.—ELIZA—Yearling filly by Vermont Boy, out of Brenda.

TERMS OF SALE.

All sums under Five Hundred Dollars, Six Months credit and Twelve Months on larger sums.

The Sale will commence at Eleven O'clock.

The Cars will leave the Depot of the Tennessee and Alabama Rail Road, at a quarter and a half past Ten and convey passengers in a few hundred yards of the sale ground.

ROBT. C. FOSTER, 4th.

WESTWOOD, on Franklin Pike, 2½ miles from Nashville, July 2d, 1860.

This antebellum advertisement for the Westwood horse farm near Nashville hints at Middle Tennessee's growing role as a source for Standardbred horses. Although the wealthy concentrated on a horse's ability to race, most people simply desired a good, dependable, fast horse for the everyday needs of transportation. Standardbreds helped serve these needs. As seen in this advertisement, these horses could be bought for under $500, and Westwood provided credit terms for installment purchases. Buyers would have included locals who needed to fill a place in the stable or new arrivals who needed to travel beyond the reach of the railroad. To encourage long-distance buyers, Foster also noted that transportation to the sale was available via the Tennessee and Alabama Railroad. (Courtesy of Gore Center.)

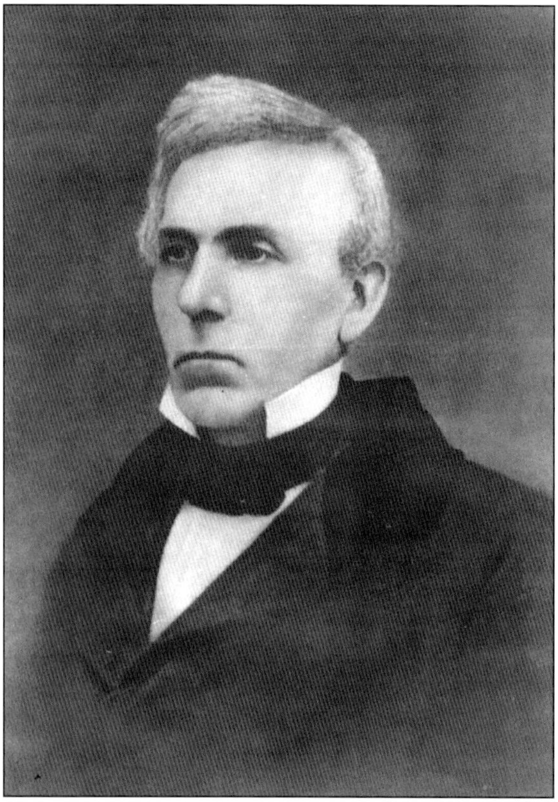

The Reverend Tolbert Fanning (1810–1874), pictured at left, was best known for his educational and religious activities. However, Fanning was also a promoter of the Morgan horse, and he supported its introduction to Middle Tennessee. Morgans originated in the mountains of Vermont as farming and riding horses. After the Civil War, Frank McGavock at Two Rivers Stock Farm in Nashville became the primary Morgan breeder in the Nashville area. David and Willie McGavock began building the mansion, pictured below, in 1859. The home was the heart of the property when Frank McGavock paid $8,000 for the Morgan stallion Ben Franklin in 1890. (Above courtesy of Gore Center; below courtesy of TSLA.)

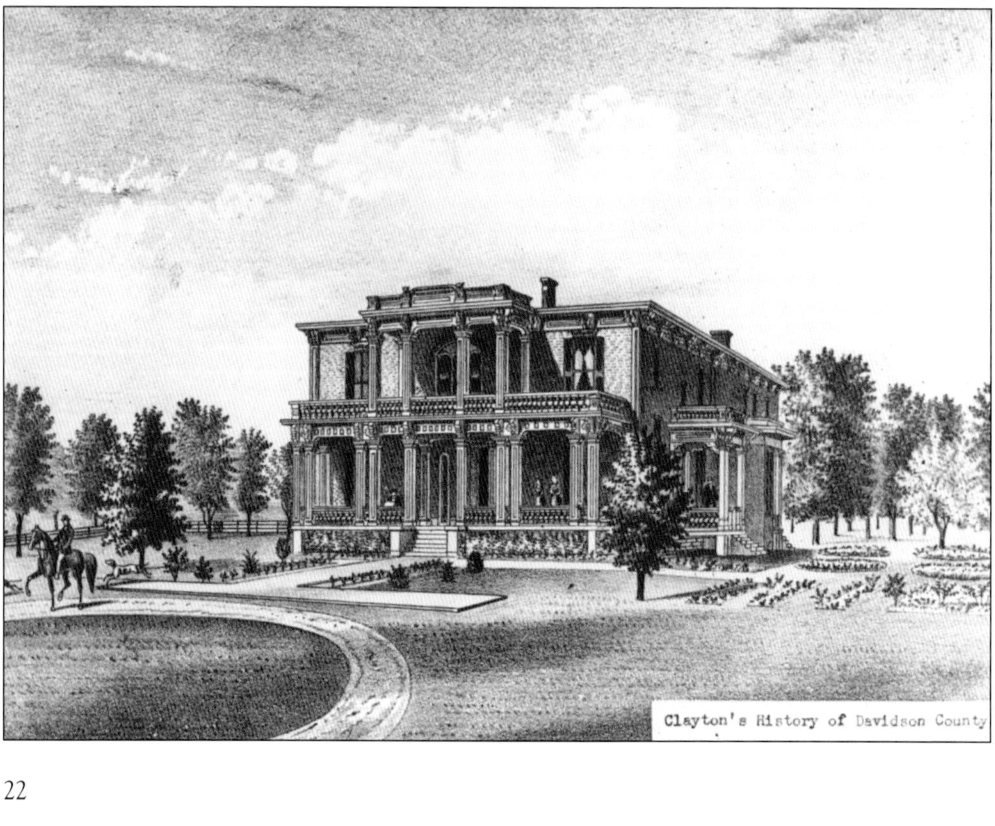

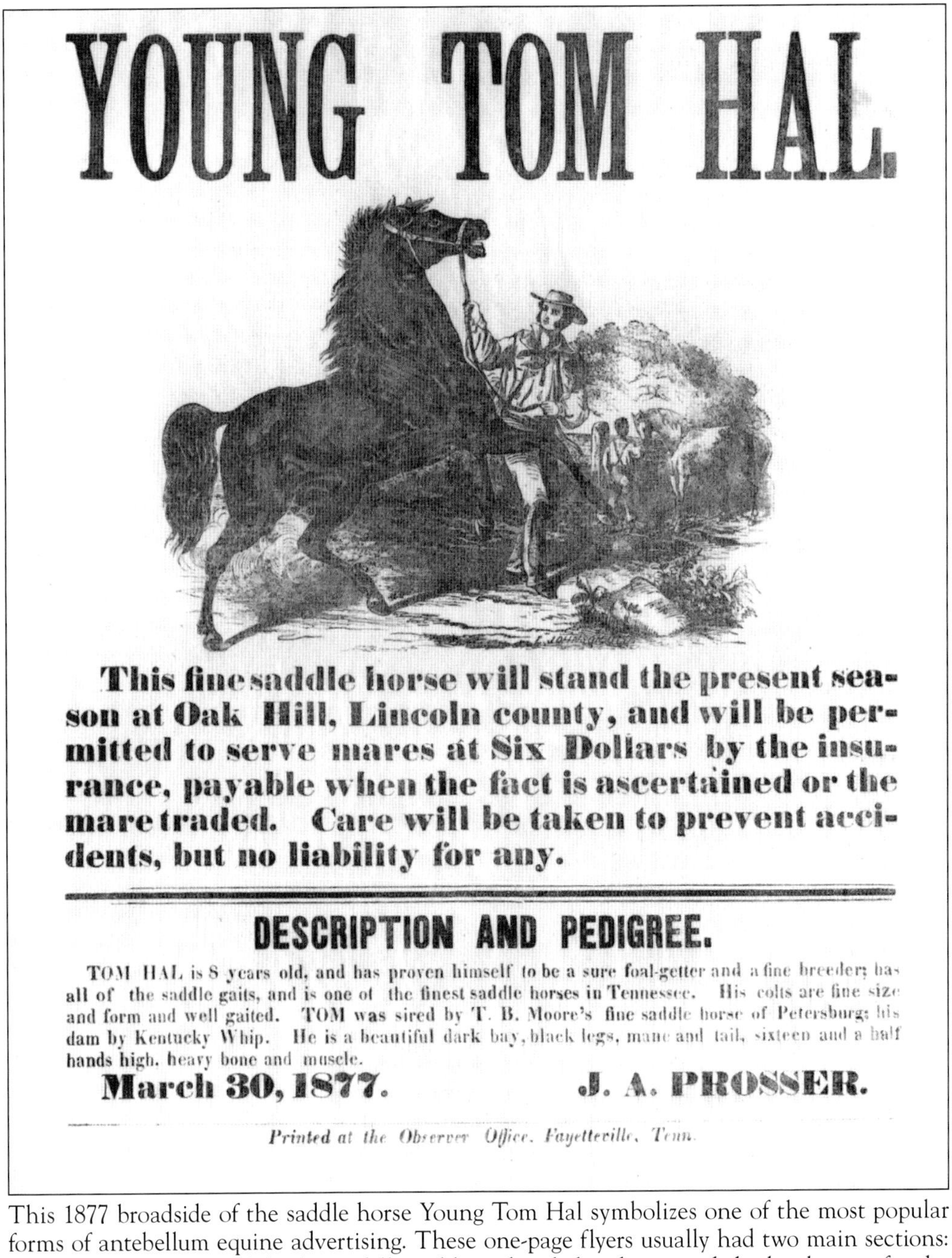

YOUNG TOM HAL.

This fine saddle horse will stand the present season at Oak Hill, Lincoln county, and will be permitted to serve mares at Six Dollars by the insurance, payable when the fact is ascertained or the mare traded. Care will be taken to prevent accidents, but no liability for any.

DESCRIPTION AND PEDIGREE.

TOM HAL is 8 years old, and has proven himself to be a sure foal-getter and a fine breeder; has all of the saddle gaits, and is one of the finest saddle horses in Tennessee. His colts are fine size and form and well gaited. TOM was sired by T. B. Moore's fine saddle horse of Petersburg; his dam by Kentucky Whip. He is a beautiful dark bay, black legs, mane and tail, sixteen and a half hands high, heavy bone and muscle.

March 30, 1877. **J. A. PROSSER.**

Printed at the Observer Office, Fayetteville, Tenn.

This 1877 broadside of the saddle horse Young Tom Hal symbolizes one of the most popular forms of antebellum equine advertising. These one-page flyers usually had two main sections: a physical description of the horse followed by a detailed pedigree and the legal terms for the breeding contract. In this case, Young Tom Hal was a young but experienced stallion of slightly above-average height, with a well-proportioned body. His pedigree was extended two generations, and interested mare owners would pay $6 for the season. If the mare did not conceive, then the fee would be waived. Because of the extra care that must be taken to manage a breeding stallion, he would remain at his home stable, and mares would be taken to stay for a period of a few days to a few weeks at the stallion's farm. By the early 1880s, this type of advertising had passed out of vogue as detailed catalogs became more popular. (Courtesy of TSLA.)

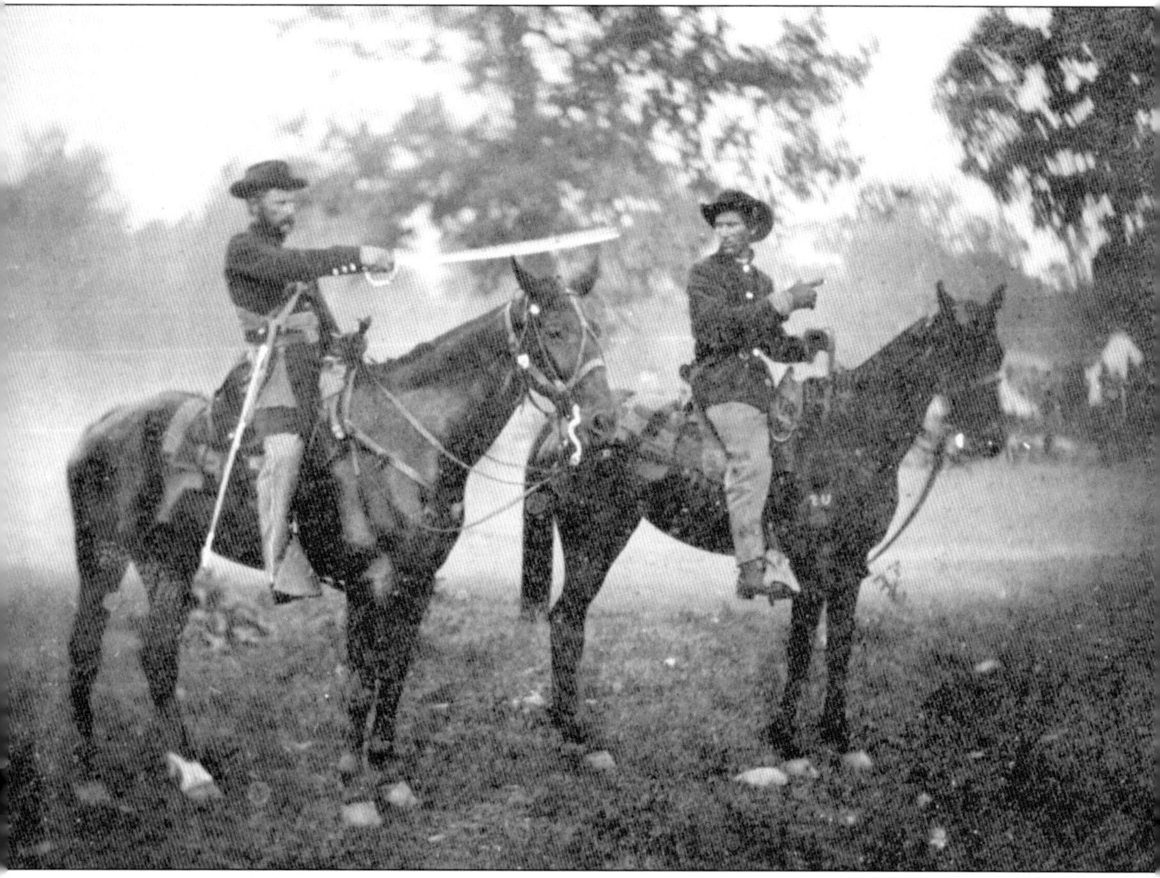

This rare Civil War–era photograph shows Capt. George Grisham, Company I, 8th Tennessee U.S. Cavalry, giving instructions to Lt. Henry Jackson, Company E, 9th Tennessee U.S. Cavalry. The tintype was taken in Gallatin on June 27, 1864. Horses were very important to the functioning of the military well into the 20th century. During the Civil War, Confederate cavalry men often bragged that their Southern-bred horses performed better in battle than their Northern counterparts. But little of this mattered as the Union army increasingly occupied Southern states during the course of the war and confiscated or bought Southern horses. Injuries sustained in battle, fatigue, and malnutrition killed an estimated one million horses and mules between 1861 and 1865. It took over a decade for the South to replenish its stock of horses to prewar levels. (Courtesy of Tennessee State Museum.)

Two

1865–1906

By 1886, Middle Tennessee reemerged as a major breeding ground for Thoroughbred as well as Standardbred horses, especially pacers. These Tennessee breeders often operated larger and more specialized farms than those found in the region prior to the Civil War. In Sumner and Davidson Counties, Thoroughbred breeding was once again in full swing at studs such as Fairvue and Belle Meade. Ewell Farm in Spring Hill was one of the first to introduce Jersey cattle and harness-racing horses to the South. And new Standardbred ventures, such as Hermitage Stud in Nashville, opened as harness racing grew in popularity.

Fortunately, there exists a rich photographic record of this reemergence of horse breeding. These Tennessee breeders were eager to celebrate—and record for posterity—their success in producing horses that once again graced major racing venues in the country. However, these ventures were fairly short-lived. A number of factors led to the decline of Thoroughbred and Standardbred breeding in Middle Tennessee at the end of the 19th century. The financial panic of 1893, geographical separation from the wealthy New York tracks and markets, the Tennessee anti-betting law of 1906, sprawling suburban development, and the passing of a generation of influential horse breeders all contributed to this decline.

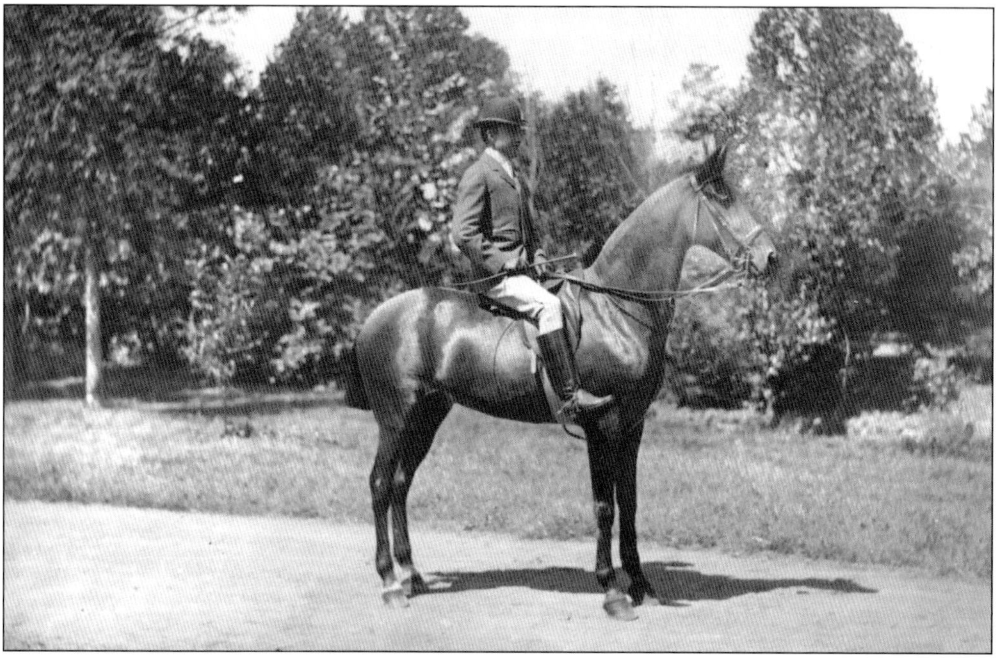

William Hicks Jackson (1835–1903), photographed here on Rennels Man, took over management of Nashville's Belle Meade Plantation from his father-in-law, William Giles Harding, by the 1880s. A former Confederate brigadier general and cavalry man, Jackson oversaw most of Belle Meade's postwar renaissance as a world-renowned Thoroughbred farm. (Courtesy of TSLA.)

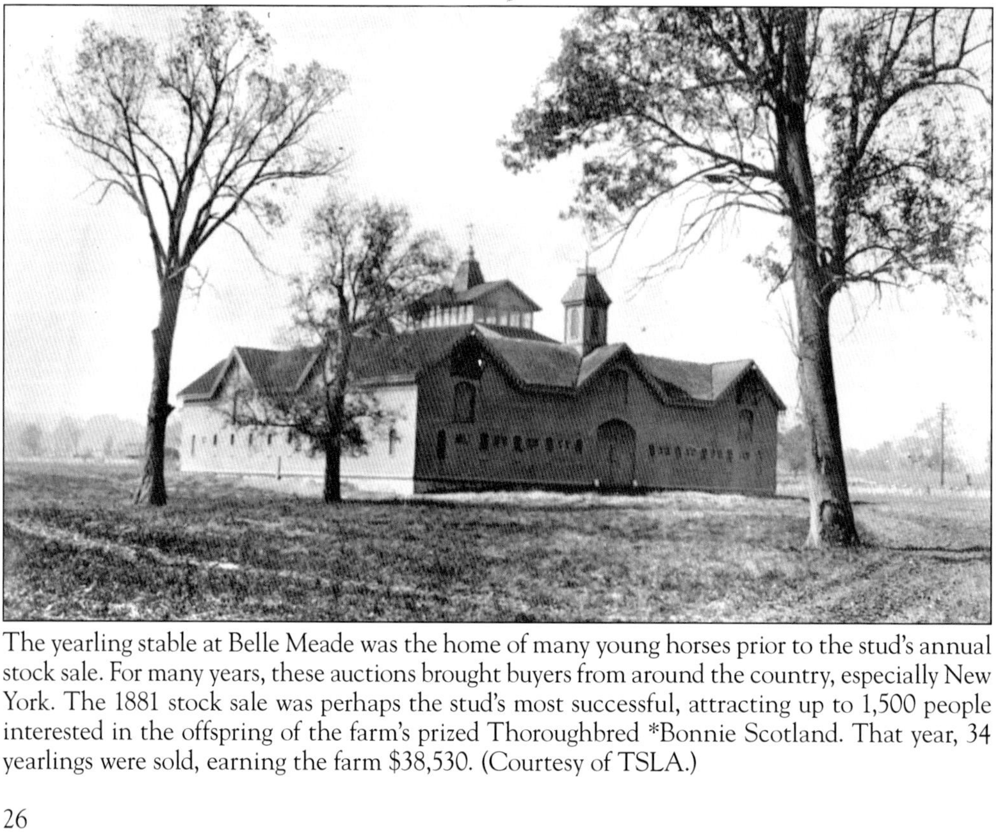

The yearling stable at Belle Meade was the home of many young horses prior to the stud's annual stock sale. For many years, these auctions brought buyers from around the country, especially New York. The 1881 stock sale was perhaps the stud's most successful, attracting up to 1,500 people interested in the offspring of the farm's prized Thoroughbred *Bonnie Scotland. That year, 34 yearlings were sold, earning the farm $38,530. (Courtesy of TSLA.)

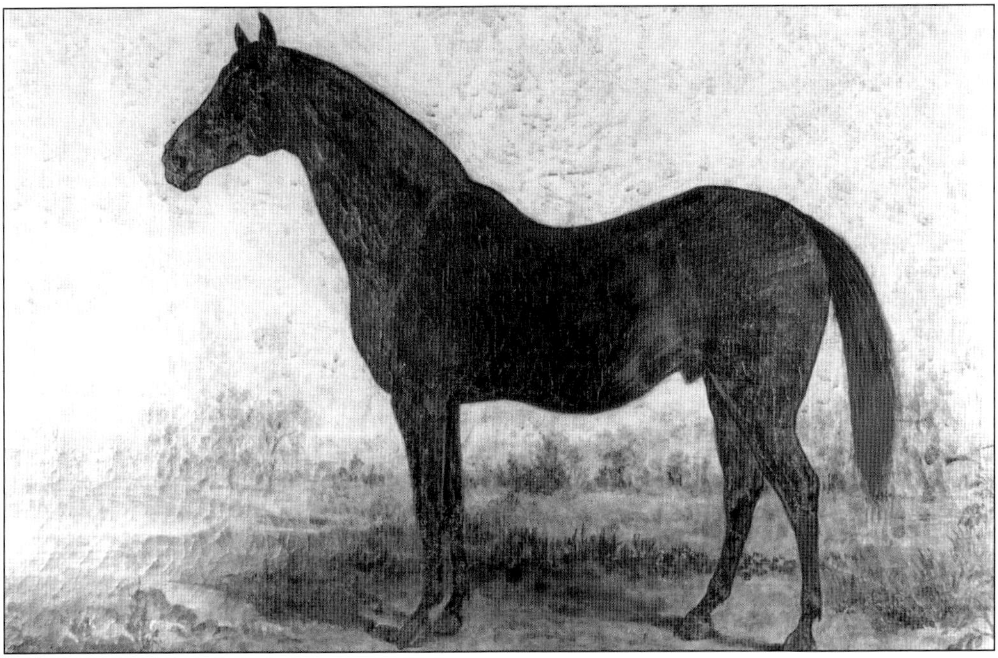

*Bonnie Scotland, depicted in this painting by Edward Troye, was foaled in England. Following an injury that prevented him from racing, he was brought to the United States to stud in 1857. Belle Meade acquired him in 1872. His offspring won an astounding 137 races in 1880, making him one of the most important Thoroughbred sires in America. (Courtesy of TSLA.)

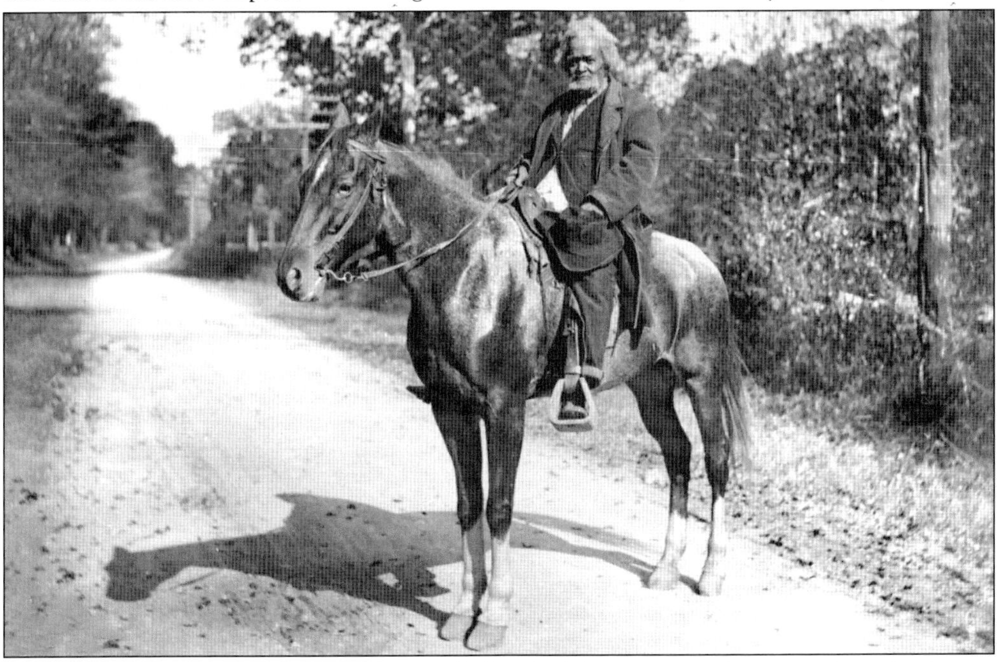

Bob Green, photographed here on Bob, was Belle Meade's primary stud groom, taking the day-to-day responsibility for the farm's stallions. Although their roles in the horse industry are frequently obscured, African American groomsmen played a vital role in the care and training of celebrated horses. (Courtesy of TSLA.)

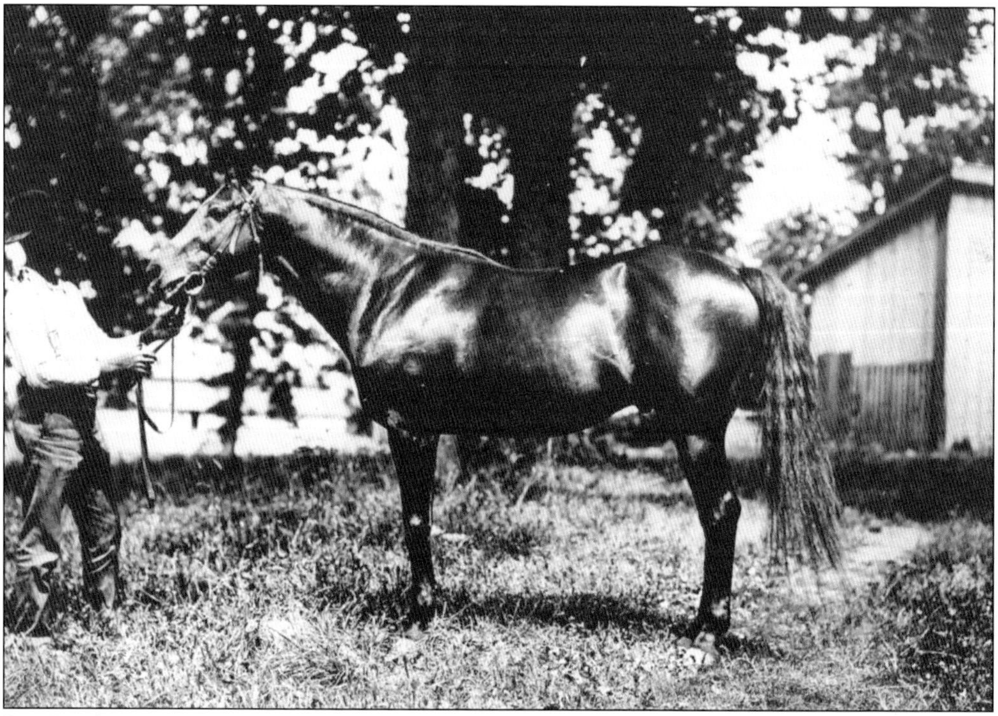

Ben Brush represents one of many successful racehorses to emerge from the *Bonnie Scotland line. His sire Bramble was sired by *Bonnie Scotland in 1875 during the latter's stint at Belle Meade. Of the 40 races he ran, he won 5, including the 1896 Kentucky Derby. (Courtesy of Gore Center.)

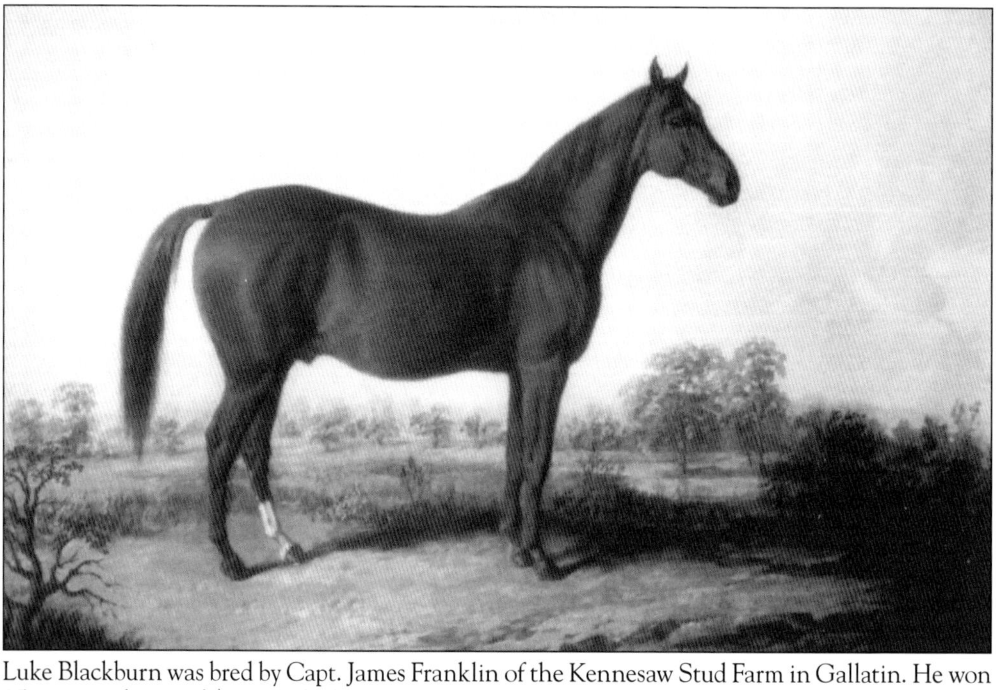

Luke Blackburn was bred by Capt. James Franklin of the Kennesaw Stud Farm in Gallatin. He won 25 races and earned $49,460 for his owners. He retired to Belle Meade to stud in 1881, replacing *Bonnie Scotland, who had died in 1880, as the farm's leading sire. (Courtesy of Gore Center.)

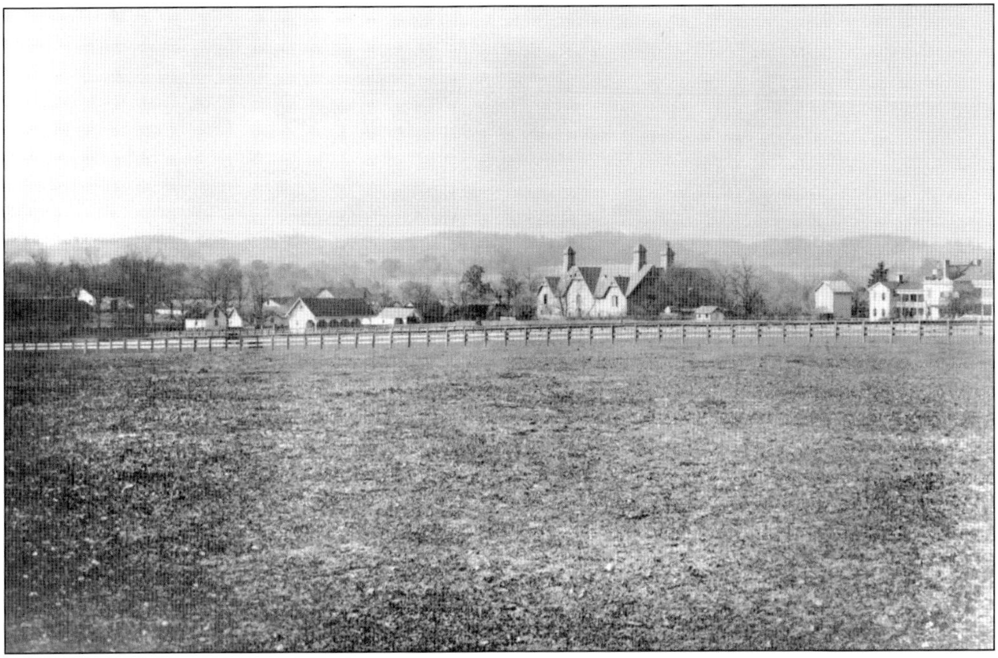

Belle Meade Plantation included many stables, outbuildings, and cross-fenced pastures to help properly care for and manage the plantation's fine bloodstock and workhorses. Not only did a well-maintained landscape impress visitors, it also reduced the frequency of accidental injuries and death to expensive livestock. (Courtesy of TSLA.)

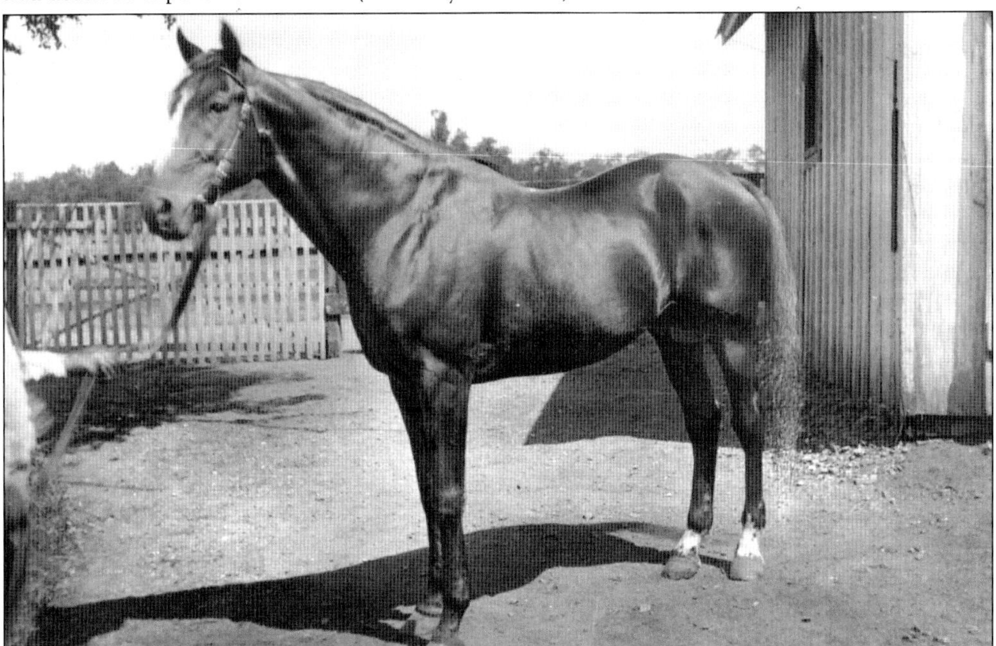

*Loyalist was a Belle Meade stallion and successful racer. Foaled in 1885, *Loyalist was one of the stud's last horses used for breeding. This photograph shows a well-balanced horse with a short back and sloping shoulder, both of which are important qualities for a racehorse. (Courtesy of TSLA.)

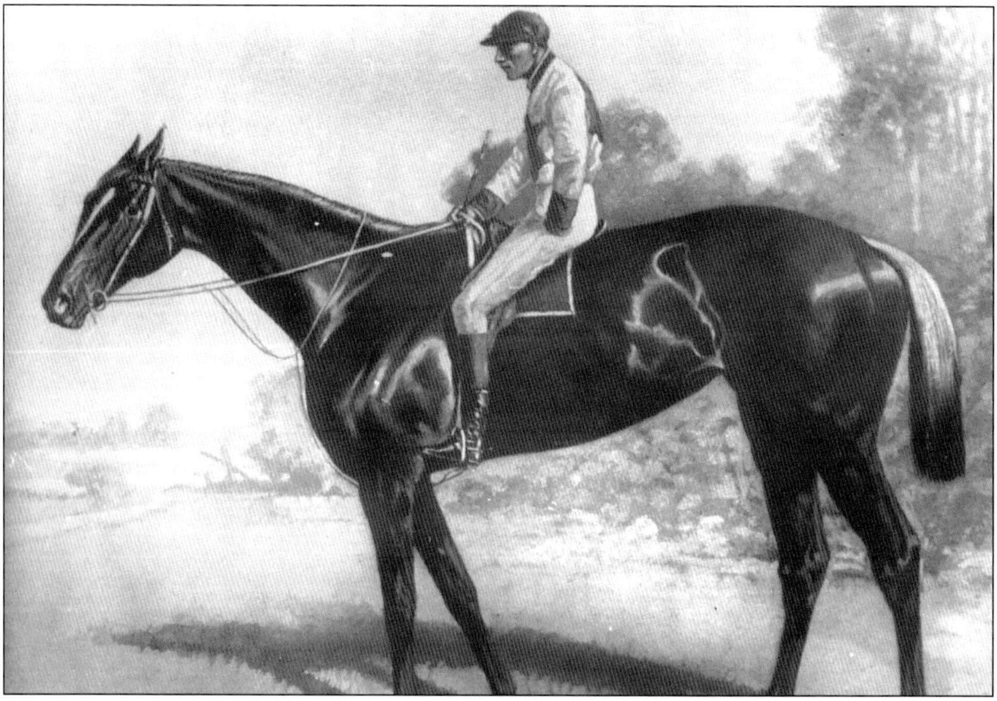

Bred by New Jersey breeder Pierre Lorillard IV, Iroquois was the first American horse to win the Epsom Derby in England. Belle Meade acquired him for $20,000 in 1887, and he quickly became the farm's leading sire. The annual Iroquois Steeplechase in Nashville is named for this horse. (Courtesy of Gore Center.)

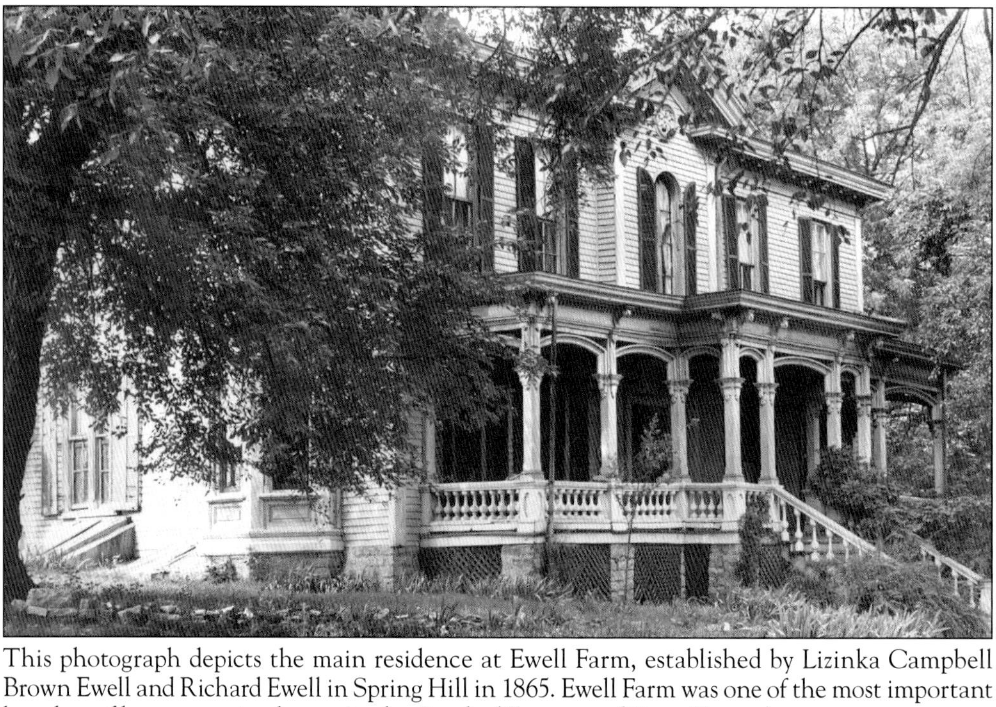

This photograph depicts the main residence at Ewell Farm, established by Lizinka Campbell Brown Ewell and Richard Ewell in Spring Hill in 1865. Ewell Farm was one of the most important breeders of harness-racing horses in the South. (Courtesy of Gore Center.)

Maj. Campbell Brown (1840–1893), Lizinka Campbell Brown Ewell's son from a previous marriage, expanded Ewell Farm into one of the region's largest livestock farms. It was one of the first to introduce Jersey cattle to the South, and it helped develop the important Hal strain of Standardbred pacers. (Courtesy of Gore Center.)

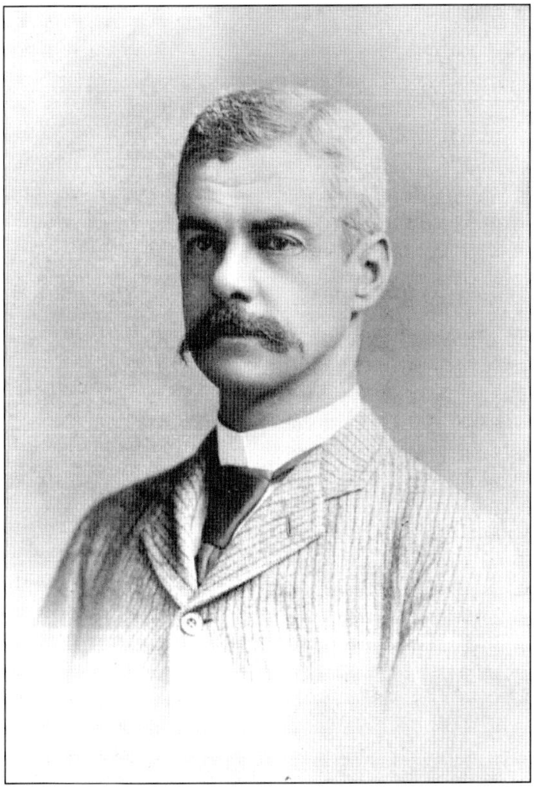

Ewell Farm built this training barn in 1883 for its increasing number of Standardbred pacers. One of these young horses was Little Brown Jug, who was promoted by John Trotwood Moore, a Columbia-based writer for the *Horse Review*. Another of the farm's famous horses was Star Pointer, the first Standardbred to trot a two-minute mile. (Courtesy of Gore Center.)

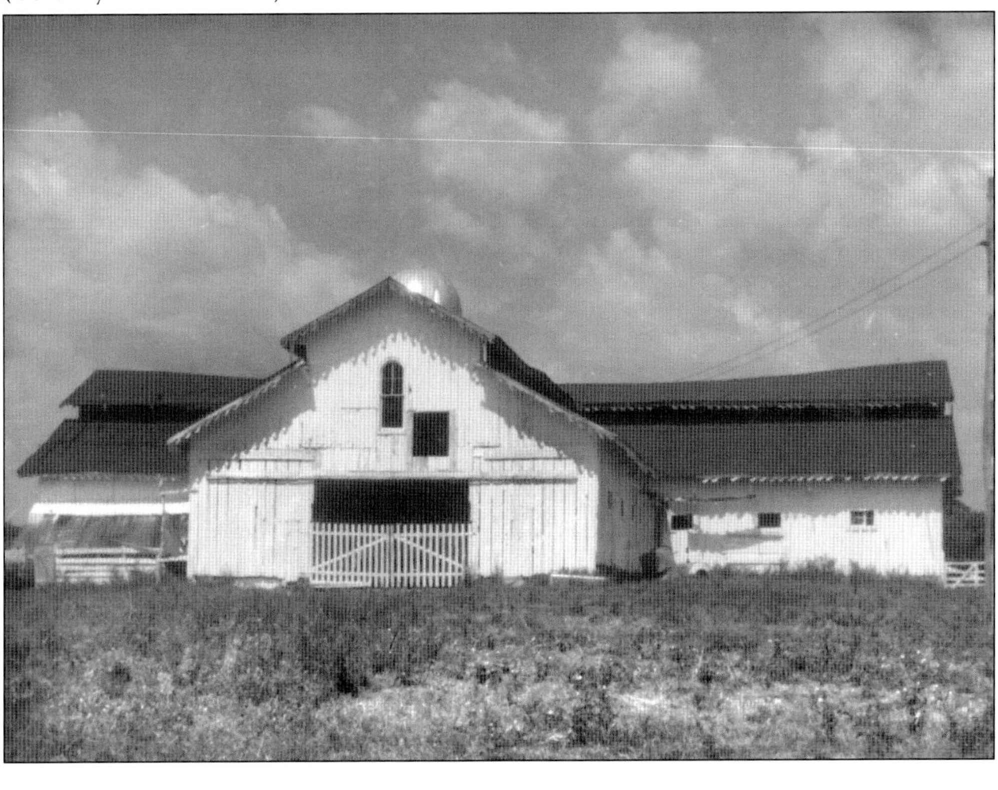

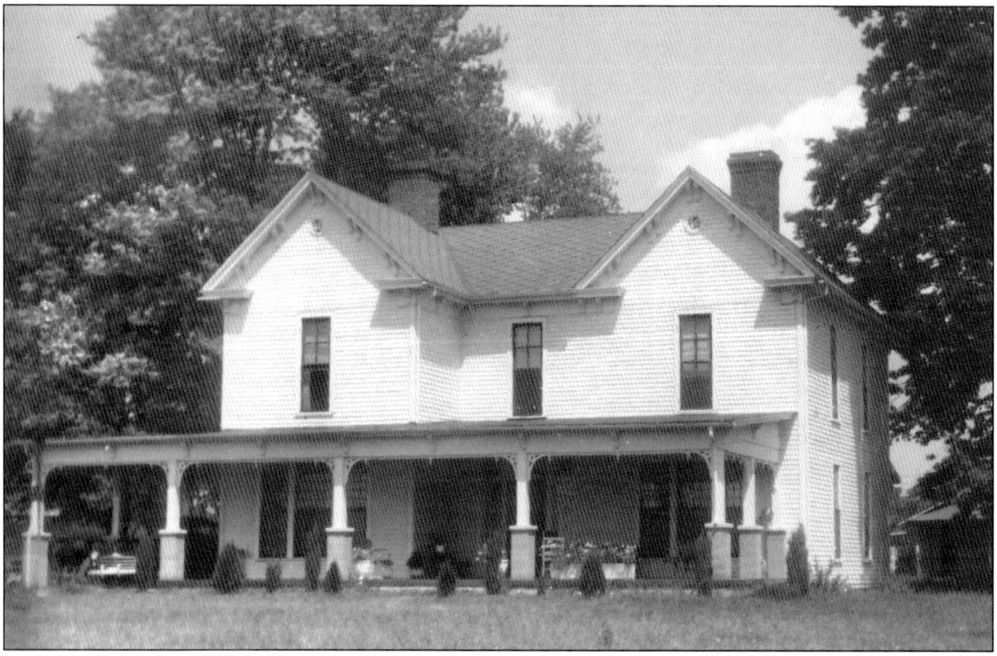

This secondary Ewell Farm house was built in 1891. E. F. "Pop" Geers, a Maury County native and legendary harness driver, lived here from 1891 to 1893. During that time, he trained some of his first national-level horses. Geers left Middle Tennessee to join the Village Stock Farm in New York, the nation's top harness stable. (Courtesy of Gore Center.)

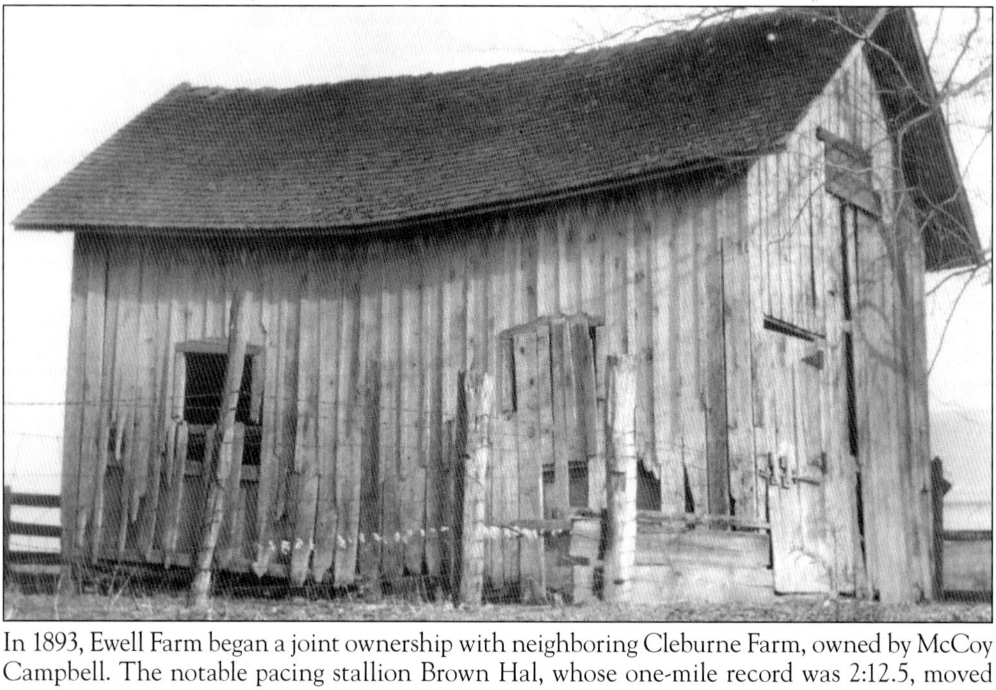

In 1893, Ewell Farm began a joint ownership with neighboring Cleburne Farm, owned by McCoy Campbell. The notable pacing stallion Brown Hal, whose one-mile record was 2:12.5, moved into this Cleburne Farm stable, which was built specifically for him. Cleburne Farm's 1893 roster also included the stallions Mercury and Actonward. This photograph was taken around 1948. (Courtesy of Gore Center.)

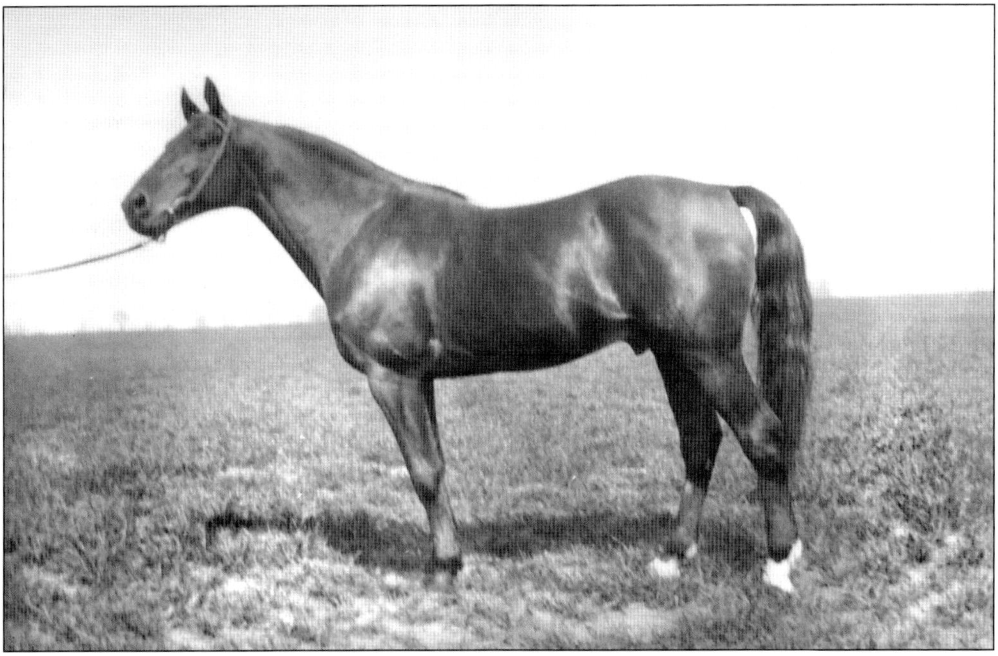

Argot Hal, whose one-mile record was 2:04.75, was sired by Brown Hal at Cleburne Farm. A trotting horse, he was encouraged to pace until a trainer in Memphis listened to the stallion and let him trot—and trot he did. In 1911, the stallion went undefeated in 11 races. (Courtesy of Gore Center.)

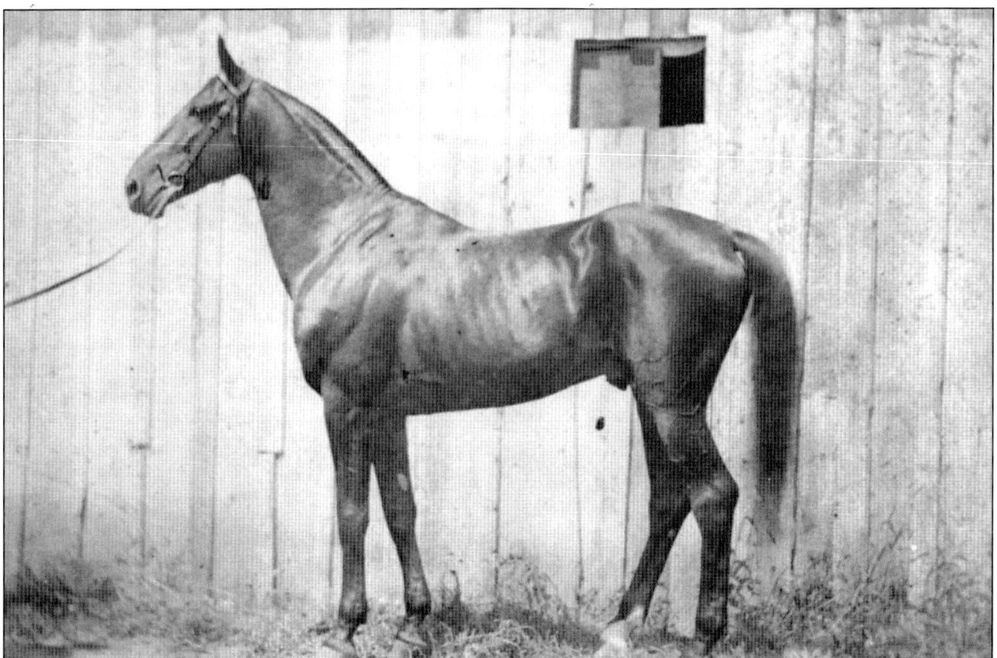

Blackwood Jr., called the "Iron Horse of Tennessee," sired several horses raised in the Pulaski area. He trotted from 1874 to 1877, winning 15 races. His offspring included five trotters and one pacer with one-mile records under 2:50. (Courtesy of Gore Center.)

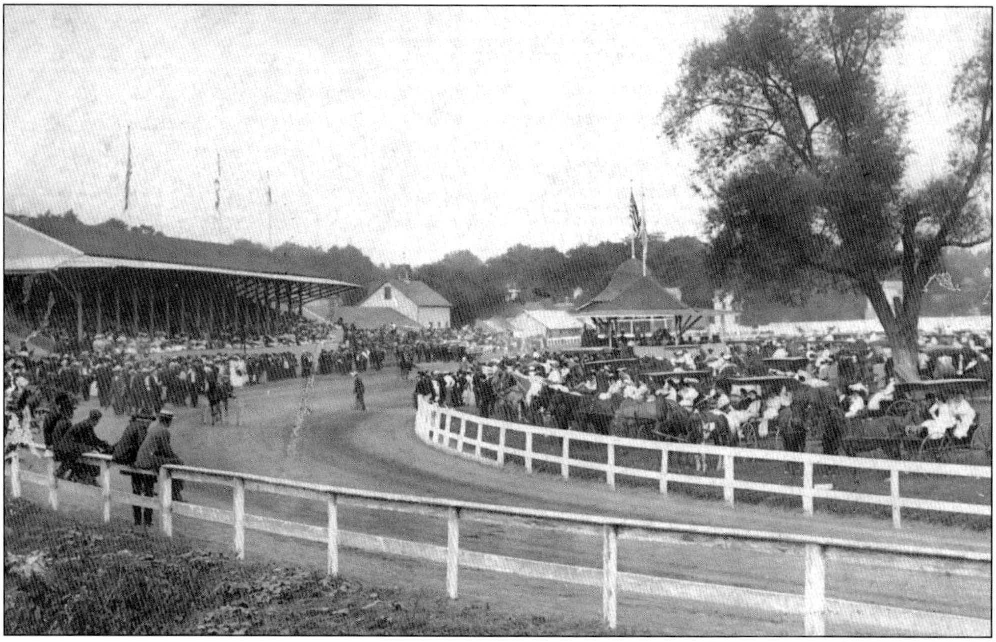

This late-19th-century photograph of a horse racing track, located in Fayetteville, serves as a reminder of the popularity of horse racing among Middle Tennesseans. For those who had nothing to do with the large tracks in Nashville, they could attend the 30 tracks estimated to be in the region around 1900. (Courtesy of TSLA.)

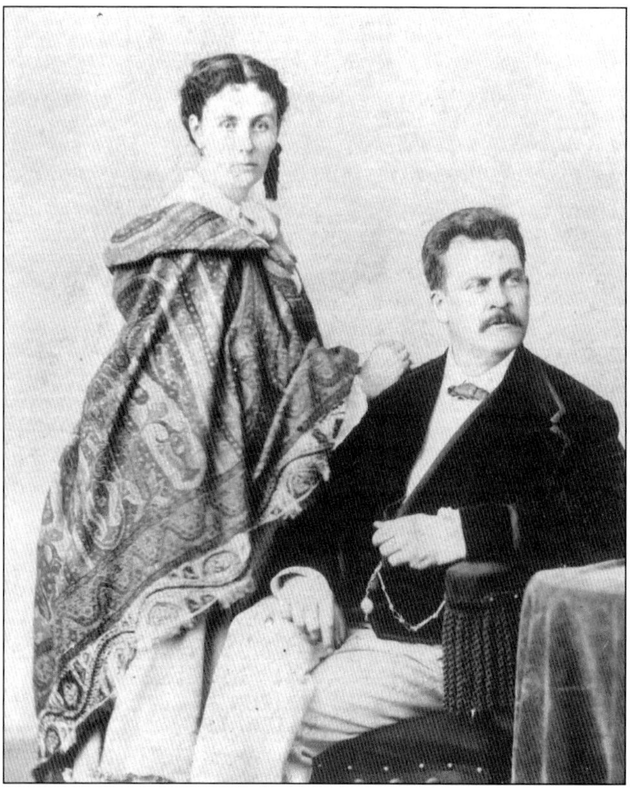

Pictured here are Charles and Ann Jane Reed of New York City. In 1882, they purchased the 2,000-acre Fairvue Plantation, located in Gallatin, Tennessee, from Adelicia Acklen for $50,000. The Reeds renamed the property Fairview. (Courtesy of Gore Center.)

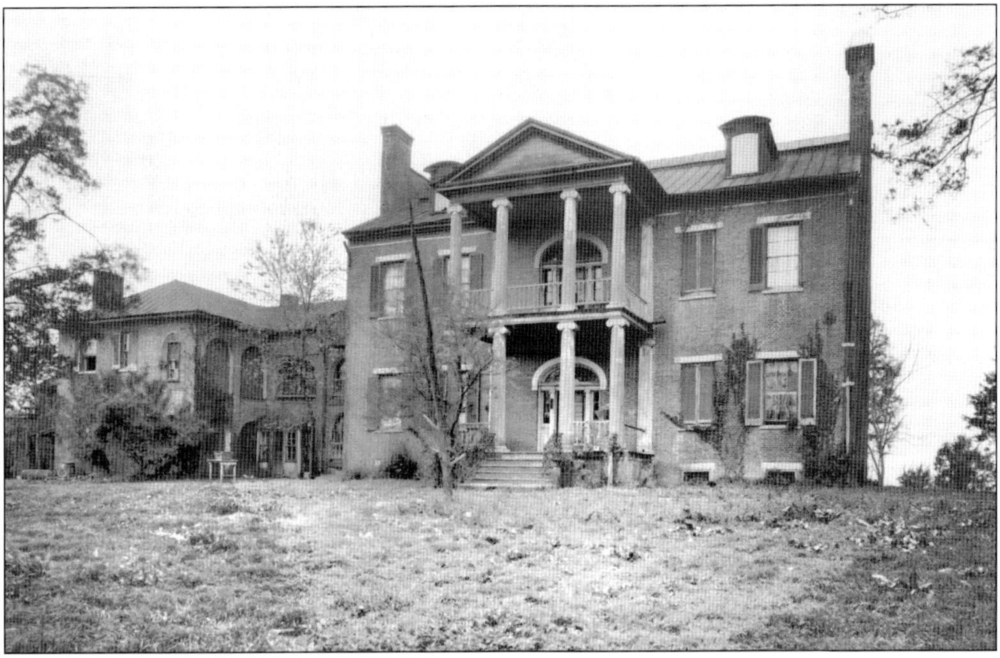

The mansion at Fairview Plantation, seen in this late-19th-century photograph, was built in 1833 by Isaac Franklin. The Reeds spent a reported $200,000 to update the home and establish Fairview as a Thoroughbred stud. The Reeds owned the property until around 1909, when their finances had dwindled to a small fraction of their previous wealth. (Courtesy of Gore Center.)

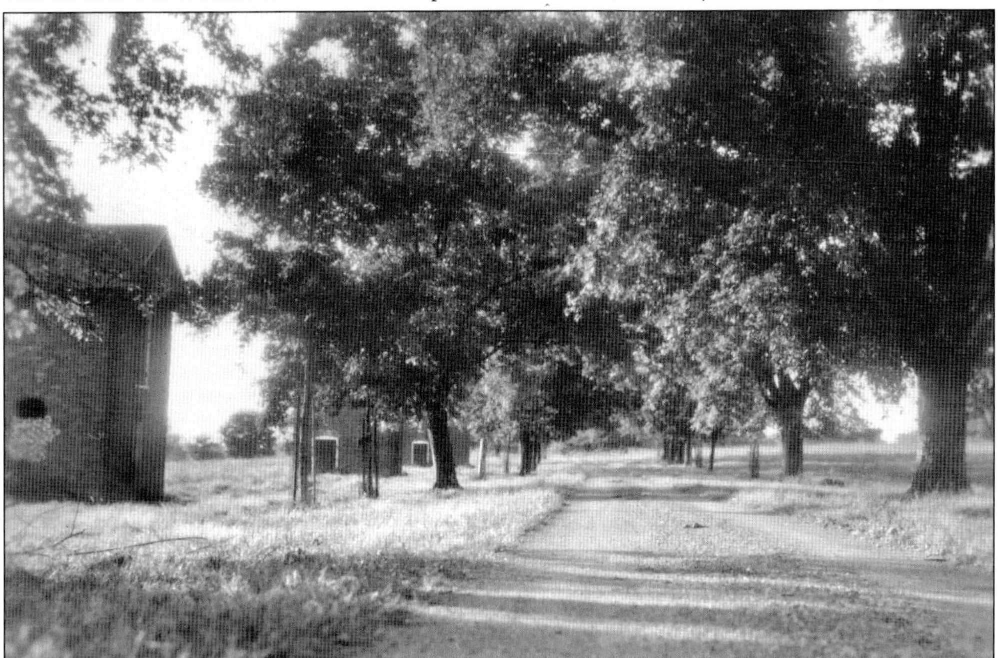

Broadway, the main road leading to the mansion, went between the individual stallion barns. The Reeds purchased the 1883 Epsom Derby winner, St. Blaise, for $100,000 and put him to stud at Fairview. (Courtesy of Gore Center.)

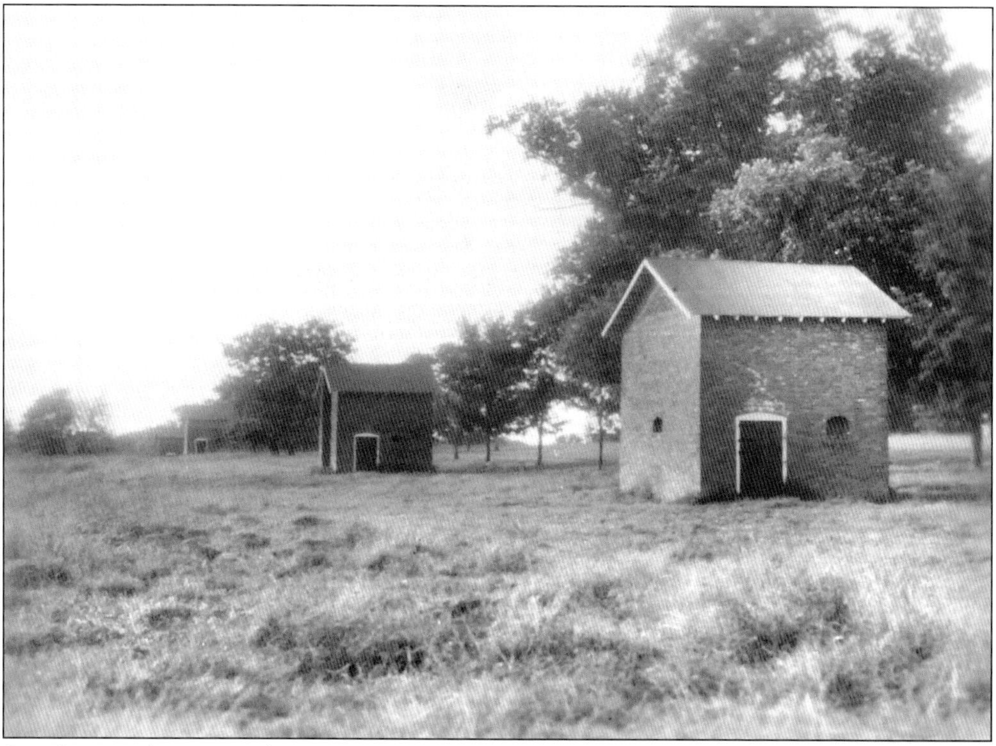

Seen here are historic and contemporary images of three of the five stallion barns that Charles Reed built at Fairview. These barns housed his Thoroughbred stallions, including Mr. Pickwick, Highlander, Fechter, Rossifer, Ill Used, and Muscovy. As can be seen in the contemporary photograph, today the stallion barns are surrounded by a housing development and a golf course. (Above courtesy of Gore Center; below photograph by April McCauley.)

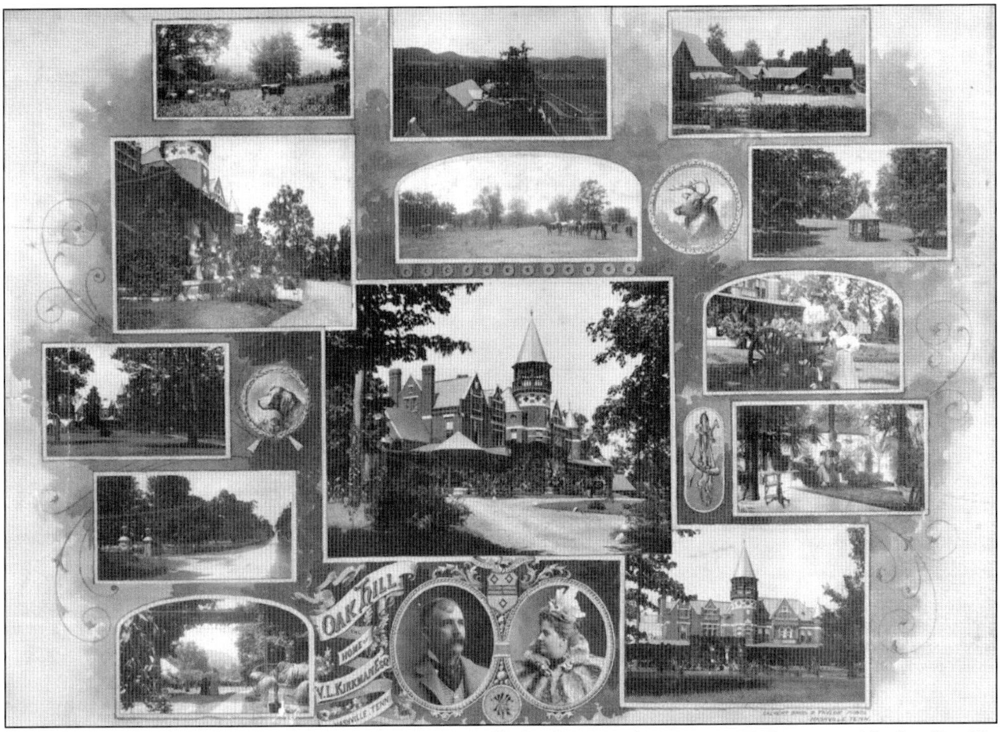

This engraving depicts multiple views of Oak Hill, the home of Van Leer Kirkman in Nashville. He served as president of the Standardbred trotting syndicate Hermitage Stud, which was established in 1887 and was located on Franklin Pike near his home south of the city. The syndicate named the stud in honor of Pres. Andrew Jackson's historic Nashville home. (Courtesy of TSLA.)

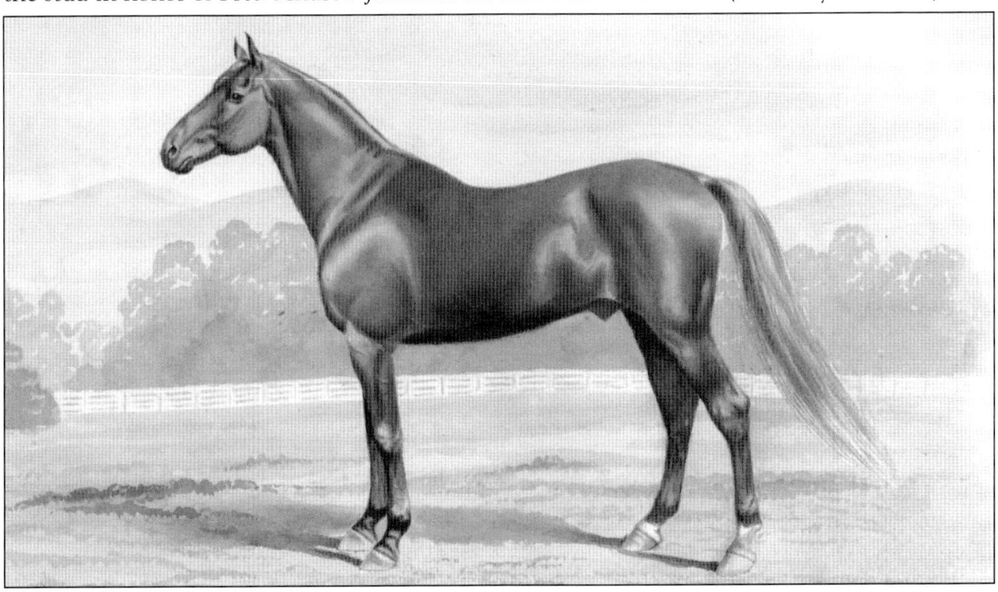

The Hermitage Stud reportedly paid $25,000 for the stallion Wedgewood, depicted in this Calvert Brothers and Taylor print. After the construction of Cumberland Park in Nashville for harness racing in 1891, the road leading from the stud to Eighth Avenue South was named Wedgewood Avenue. The road is still there today. (Courtesy of Travellers Rest Plantation and Museum.)

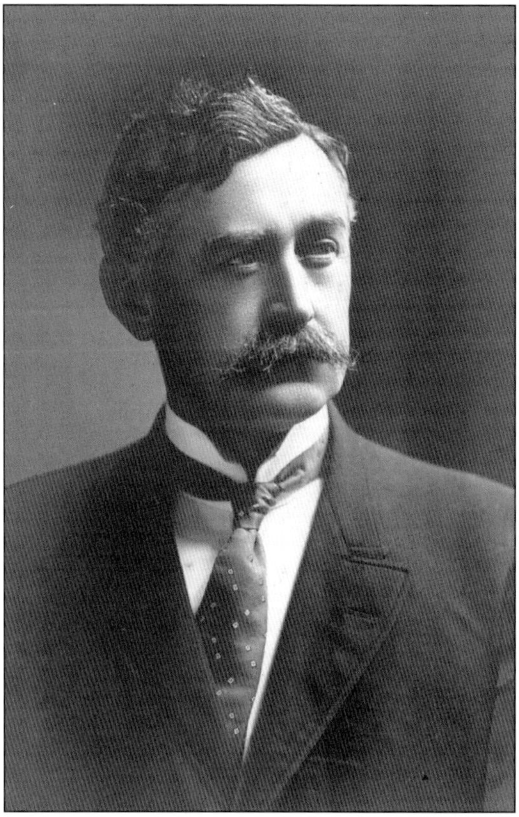

May Overton, manager of Hermitage Stud, lived at Travellers Rest, just east of the farm off Franklin Pike. He was the grandson of Judge John Overton, the original owner of Travellers Rest. Also included in the syndicate were his brothers Jesse and Robert Overton and neighbor John Thompson. (Courtesy of Gore Center.)

The office of Hermitage Stud, located in Nashville, managed the breeding seasons of its stallions and oversaw the syndicate's 1,400-acre property. This view looks west toward Franklin Road. (Courtesy of Gore Center.)

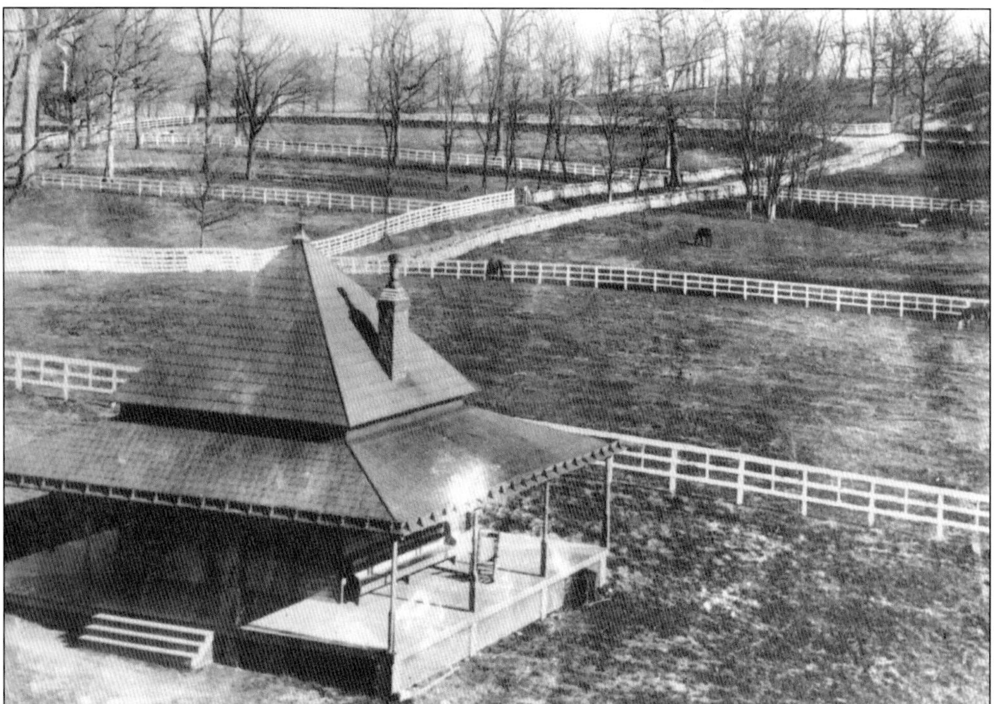

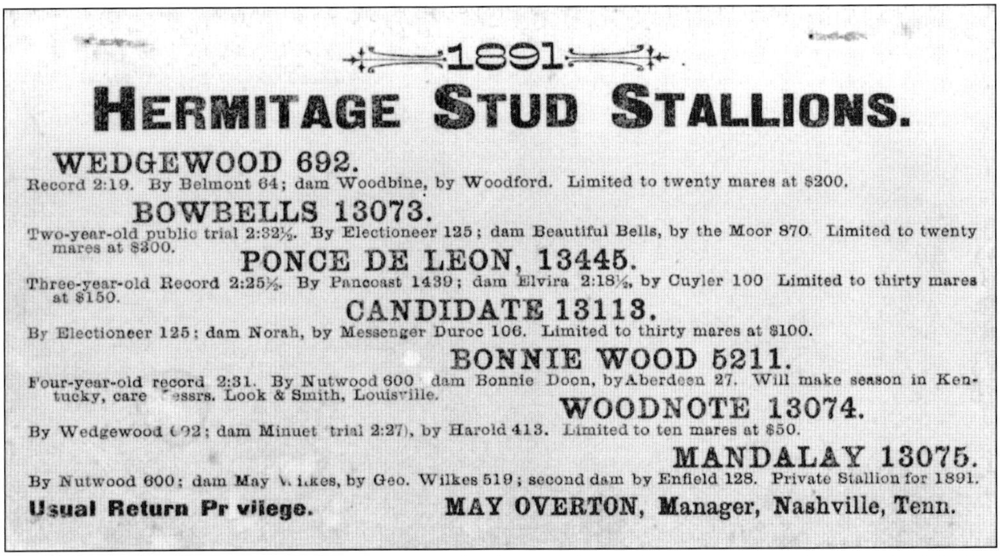
1891

HERMITAGE STUD STALLIONS.

WEDGEWOOD 692.
Record 2:19. By Belmont 64; dam Woodbine, by Woodford. Limited to twenty mares at $200.

BOWBELLS 13073.
Two-year-old public trial 2:32½. By Electioneer 125; dam Beautiful Bells, by the Moor 870. Limited to twenty mares at $300.

PONCE DE LEON, 13445.
Three-year-old Record 2:25½. By Pancoast 1439; dam Elvira 2:18¼, by Cuyler 100. Limited to thirty mares at $150.

CANDIDATE 13113.
By Electioneer 125; dam Norah, by Messenger Duroc 106. Limited to thirty mares at $100.

BONNIE WOOD 5211.
Four-year-old record 2:31. By Nutwood 600; dam Bonnie Doon, by Aberdeen 27. Will make season in Kentucky, care Messrs. Look & Smith, Louisville.

WOODNOTE 13074.
By Wedgewood 692; dam Minuet (trial 2:27), by Harold 413. Limited to ten mares at $50.

MANDALAY 13075.
By Nutwood 600; dam May Wilkes, by Geo. Wilkes 519; second dam by Enfield 128. Private Stallion for 1891.

Usual Return Privilege. MAY OVERTON, Manager, Nashville, Tenn.

This 1891 card advertises Hermitage Stud's leading stallions for the season. The card highlights distance times for the horses and lists the stud fees. (Courtesy of Gore Center.)

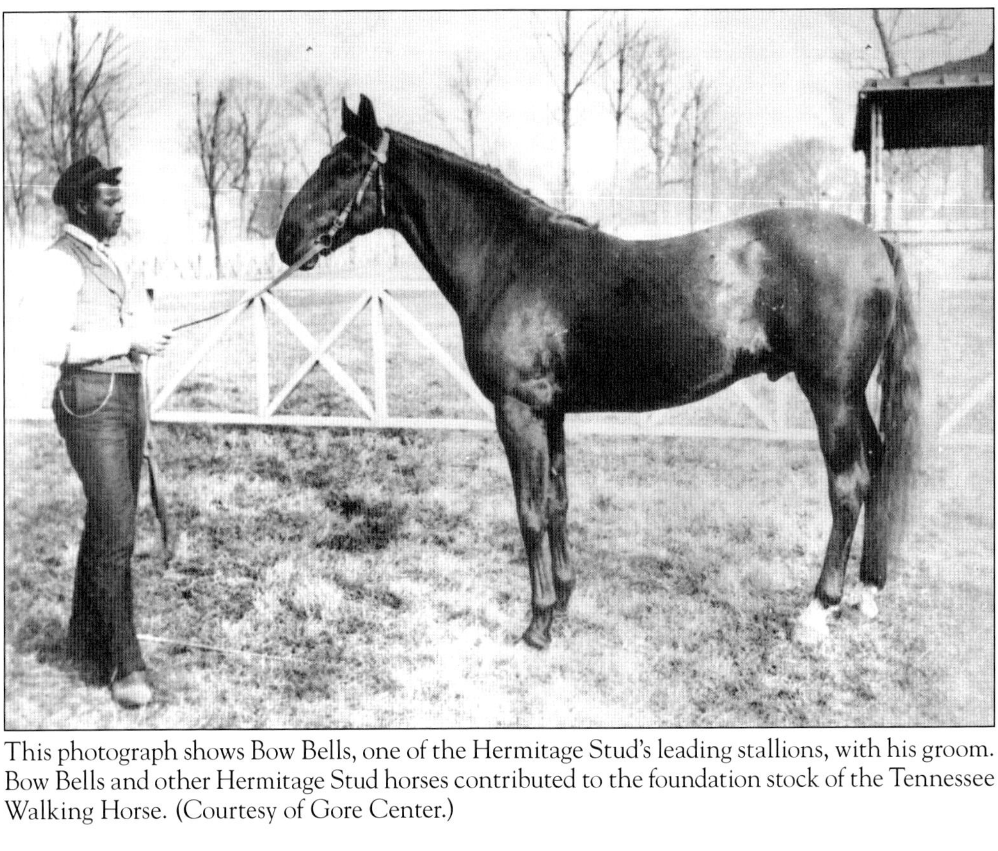

This photograph shows Bow Bells, one of the Hermitage Stud's leading stallions, with his groom. Bow Bells and other Hermitage Stud horses contributed to the foundation stock of the Tennessee Walking Horse. (Courtesy of Gore Center.)

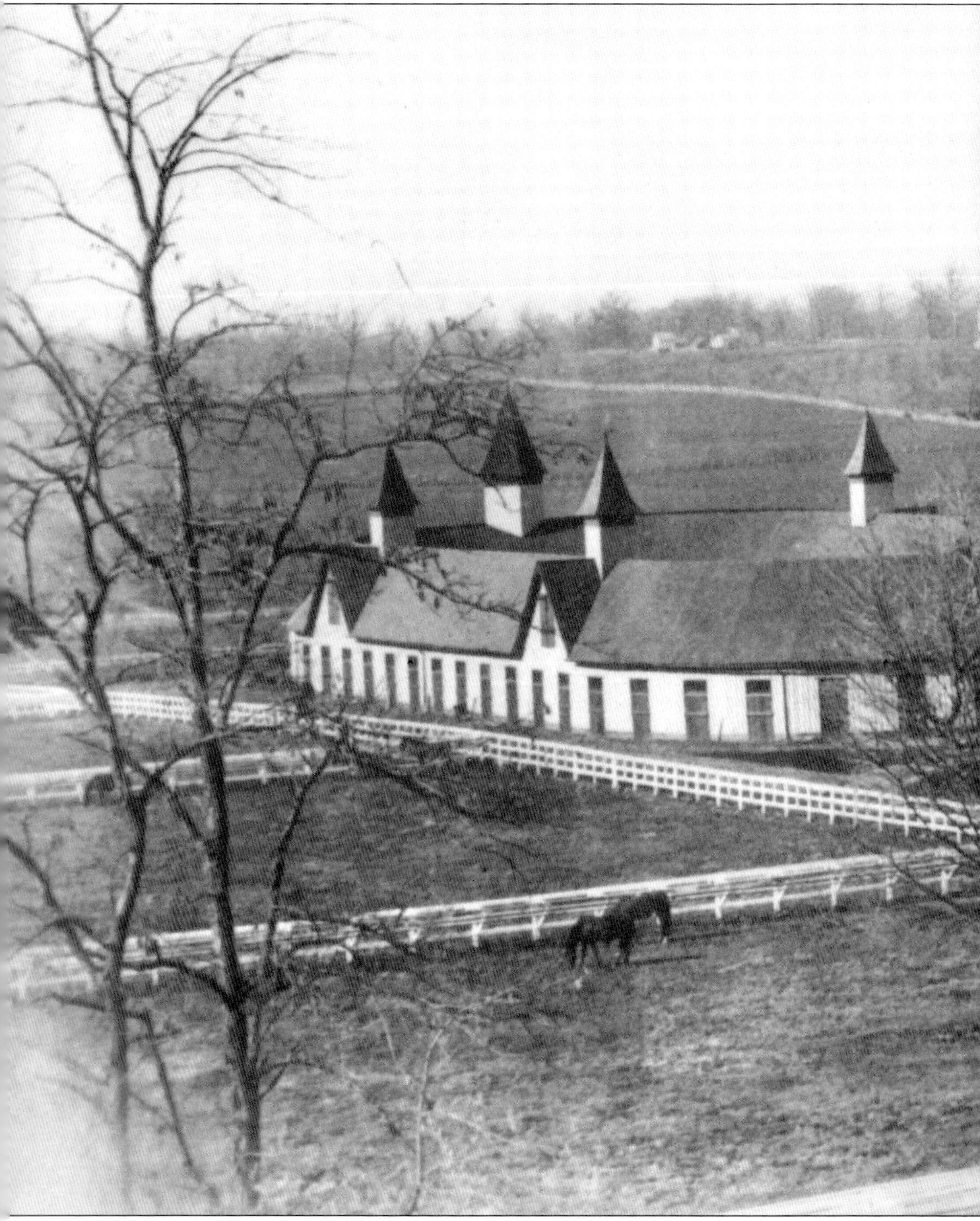

The 1,400-acre grounds of the Hermitage Stud included a covered track with 52 stalls for colts. The late 19th century marked the high point of the driving horse. Improvement of road conditions created greater demand for harness horses, which were needed to pull buggies or sulkies, than for saddle horses. The Hermitage Stud focused its resources on producing fast harness horses for

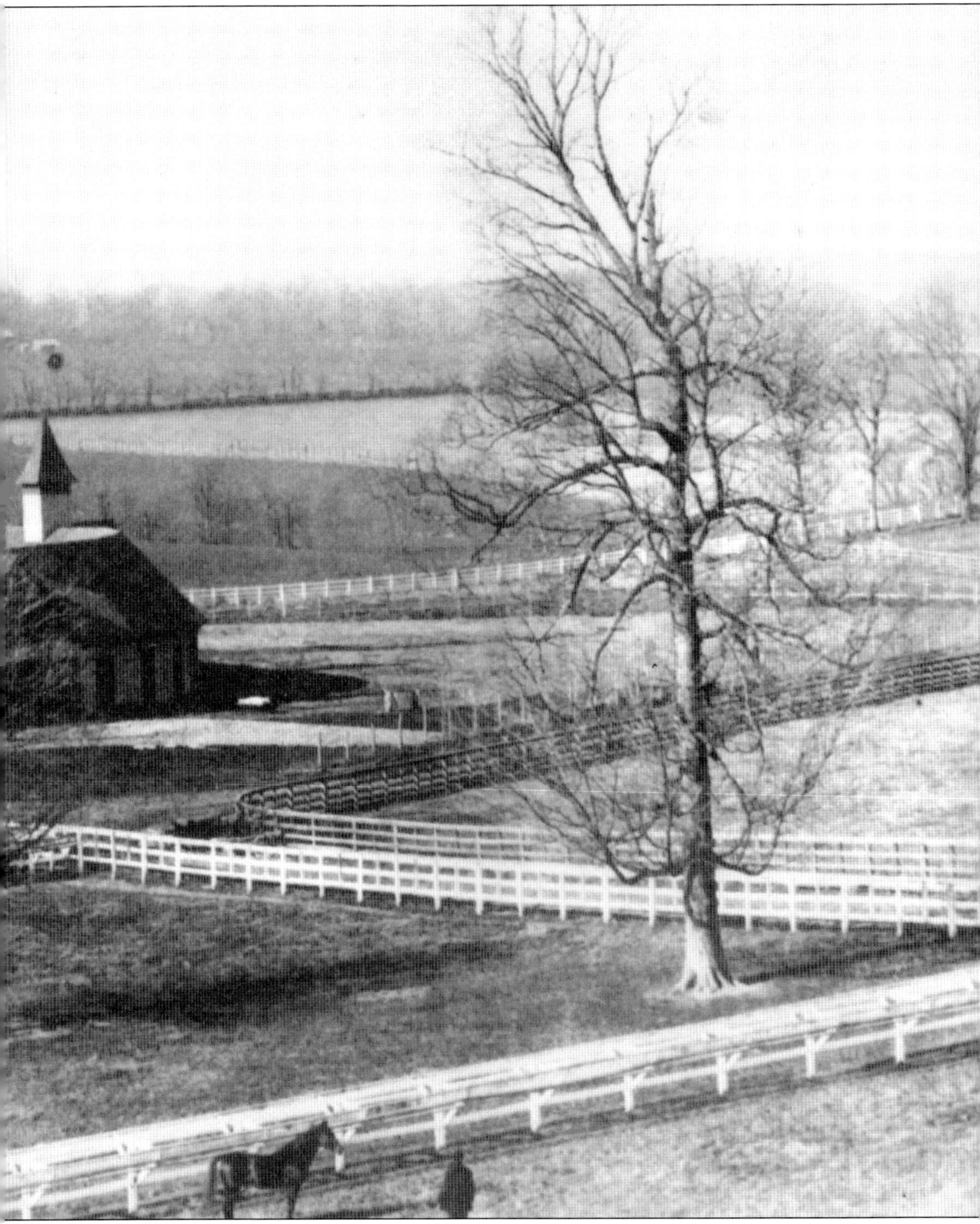

racing, but it also provided stylish road horses for private transport. The Hermitage Stud prospered until the early 20th century, when a poor market forced the syndicate to begin selling some of the property and dispersing the farm's stock. The training stable burned by 1917, removing the last traces of this once great breeding business. (Courtesy of Gore Center.)

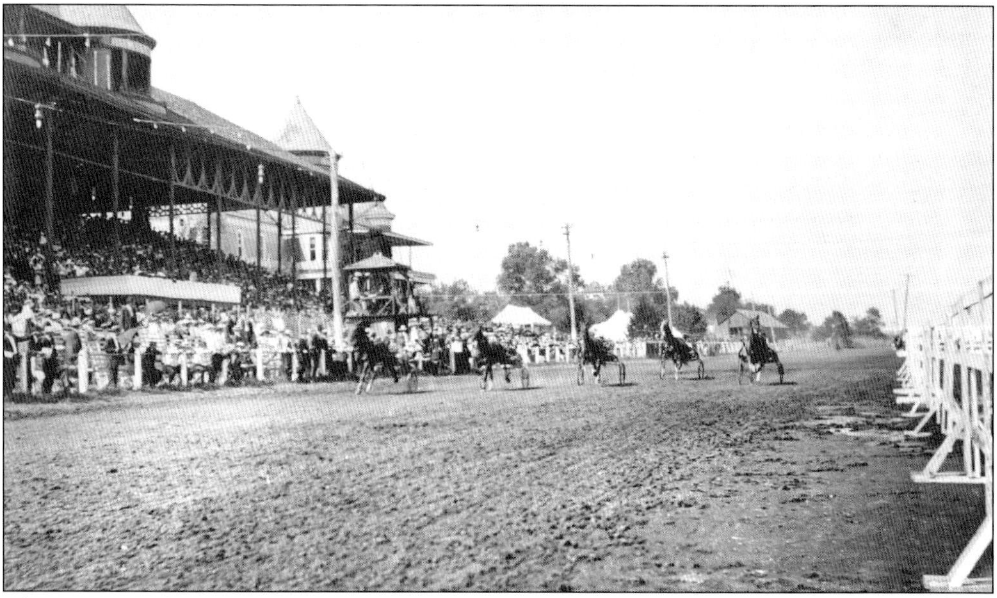

The owners of the Hermitage Stud established Cumberland Park for harness racing. The elegant club and grandstand held 7,000 spectators, and the stables could accommodate 350 horses. This *c.* 1900 photograph captures a harness race in action. Today the site is Nashville's fairgrounds. (Courtesy of Ruth Warner.)

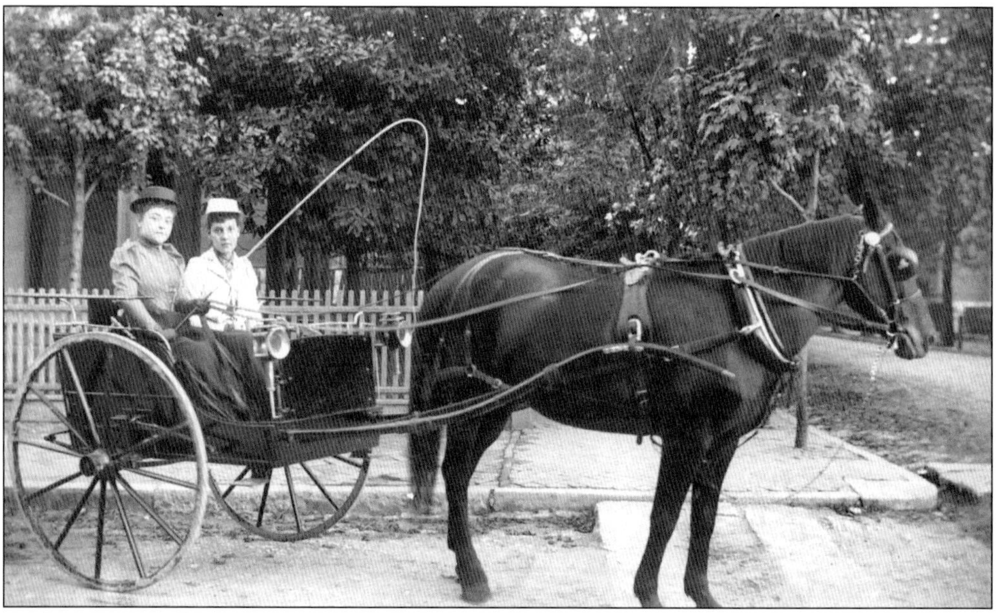

In this *c.* 1880 photograph, Murfreesboro residents Hattie Marshal and Henrietta Kendrick (whose married name was Reeves) are enjoying a socially acceptable equestrian activity: a carriage drive. Women often drove their own horses in town, and they used their buggies or carriages to make social calls. Henrietta Reeves, according to Mary Frazier of TSLA, became a "cultural and social leader in Nashville" and served as a president of the Centennial Club. (Courtesy of Gore Center.)

Maj. M. B. Kittrell (1821–1893) was a prominent Rutherford and Wilson County horse breeder. He is credited with breeding Kittrell's Tom Hal, a foundation sire of the Tennessee Walking Horse breed. (Courtesy of Gore Center.)

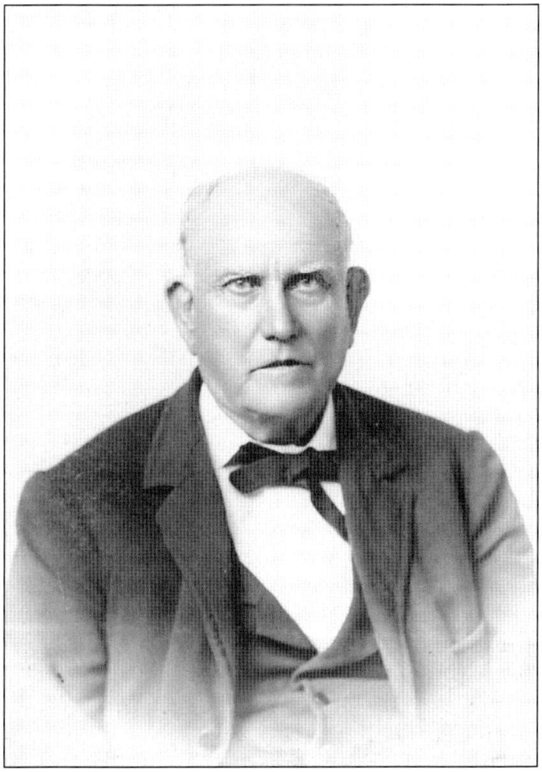

Echo, (fathered) by McCurdy 26407 by McCurdy's Hambletonian 1644 (the registration number became part of the name), is shown here outside a home in Nashville. Echo became an important contributor to the emerging Tennessee Walking Horse breed of the late 19th century. (Courtesy of Gore Center.)

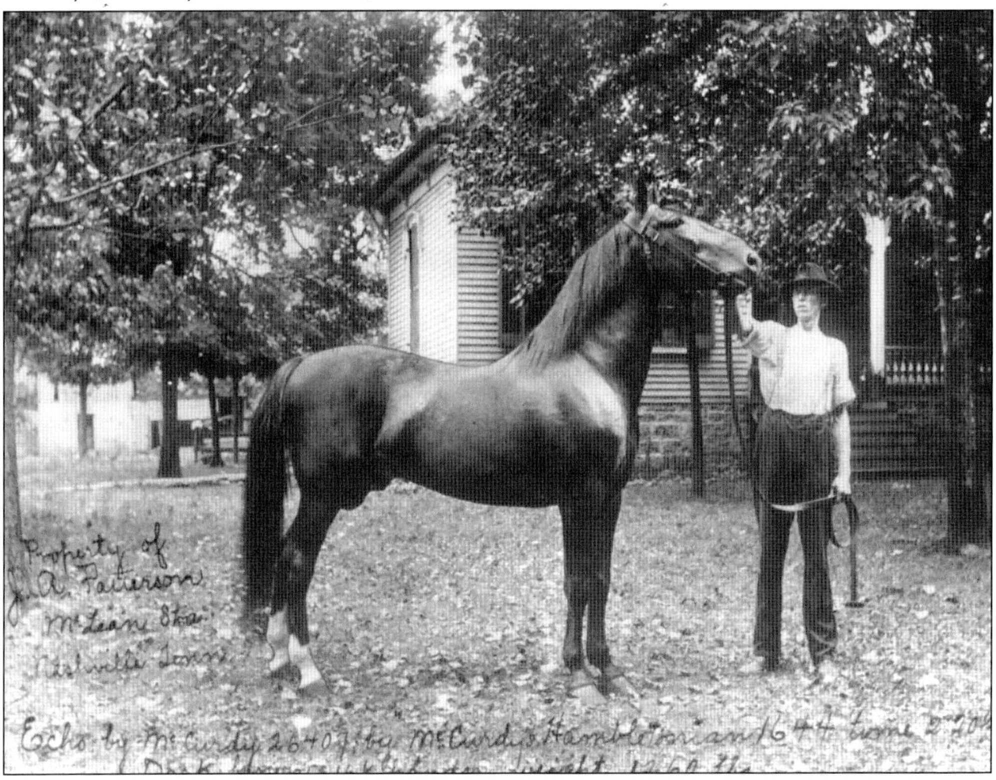

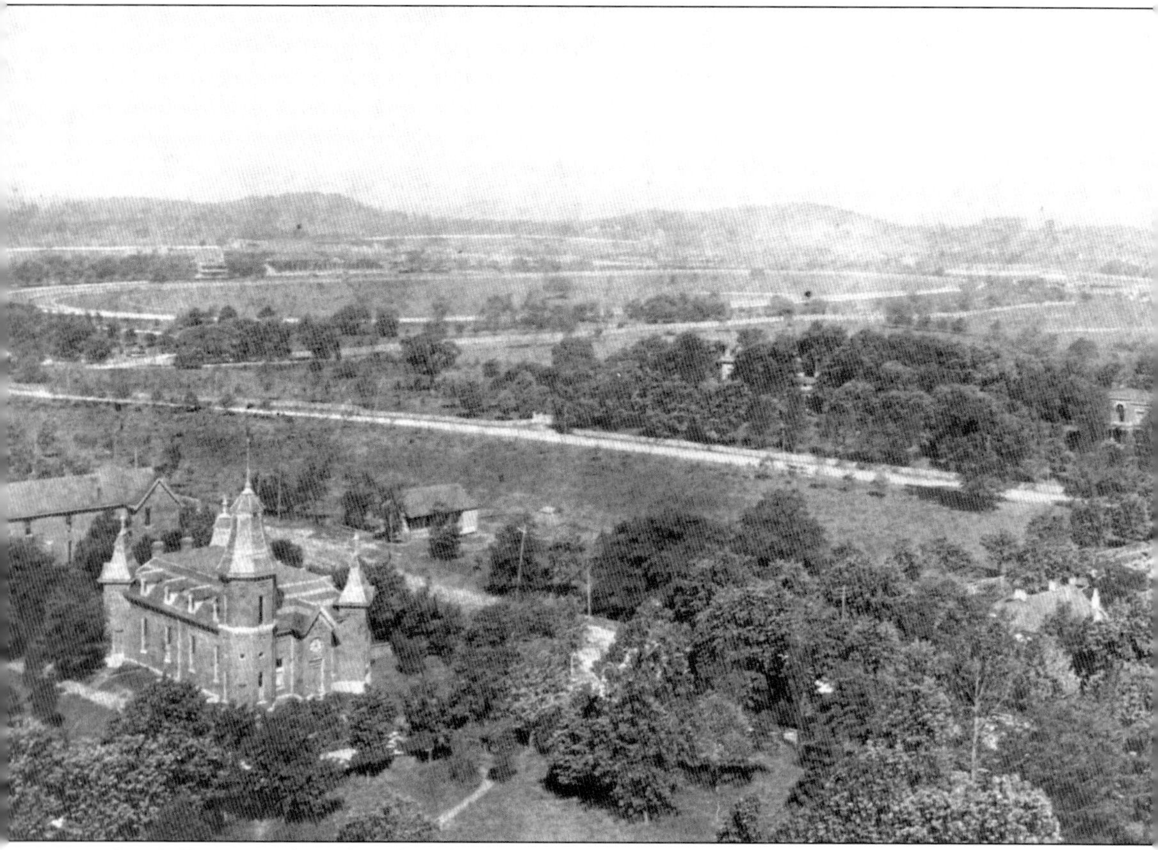

In 1887, West Side Park replaced the Island Track as Nashville's premier horse race course. But races ran at the course for only four years. The establishment of the better-equipped Cumberland Park on the southeast side of the city forced its closing. In 1896, West Side Park became the site of the Tennessee Centennial Exposition. Today it is the site of the Parthenon and Centennial Park. (Courtesy of TSLA.)

Three

Workhorses and Mules

In addition to using horses and mules as a means of transportation, the early settlers of Middle Tennessee also used them to carry loads, to pull wagons and plows, to haul logs out of cleared land, and to perform many other vital chores associated with an agricultural economy. The cost of a workhorse or mule is much more than its initial purchase price. These animals require harnesses, shelter, and food, which resulted in a significant investment for most Middle Tennesseans in the late 18th and early 19th centuries.

As with pleasure horses, well-bred, higher-quality workhorses and mules perform better and longer. In the mid-19th century, Middle Tennessee breeders began to concentrate on producing mules with excellent conformation (the shape and balance of the body and limbs) to fill this need, while their northern counterparts began instead to import European draft horses.

By the end of the 19th century, Middle Tennessee (Columbia, in particular) had emerged as a nationally recognized leader of mule production. The Boer War and World War I resulted in a boom for Middle Tennessean mule breeders. Most militaries continued to use mules for transport and as pack animals. Mules often carried hundreds of pounds of weapons and supplies into combat. In World War I, the American Expeditionary Force even issued gas masks to its horses and mules to help them survive on the front lines. In addition, a combination of high-quality stock, economic uncertainties (including the Depression), and plentiful supply resulted in the continued use of mules in Middle Tennessee agriculture.

After World War II, the use of workhorses and mules declined significantly. Reasons for this decline included the low cost of tractors, continued competition from Missouri mule breeders, increased land prices (owning mules and workhorses usually required significant acreage devoted to grazing rather than to crop production), and the almost complete transformation of the Tennessee Walking Horse from a workhorse to pleasure and show horse.

By the 1990s, Middle Tennessean mule breeders once again produced for a national market, including Amish farmers in the Northeast, hunting and pack outfitters in the West, and, recently, prospective buyers for the U.S. military in Afghanistan.

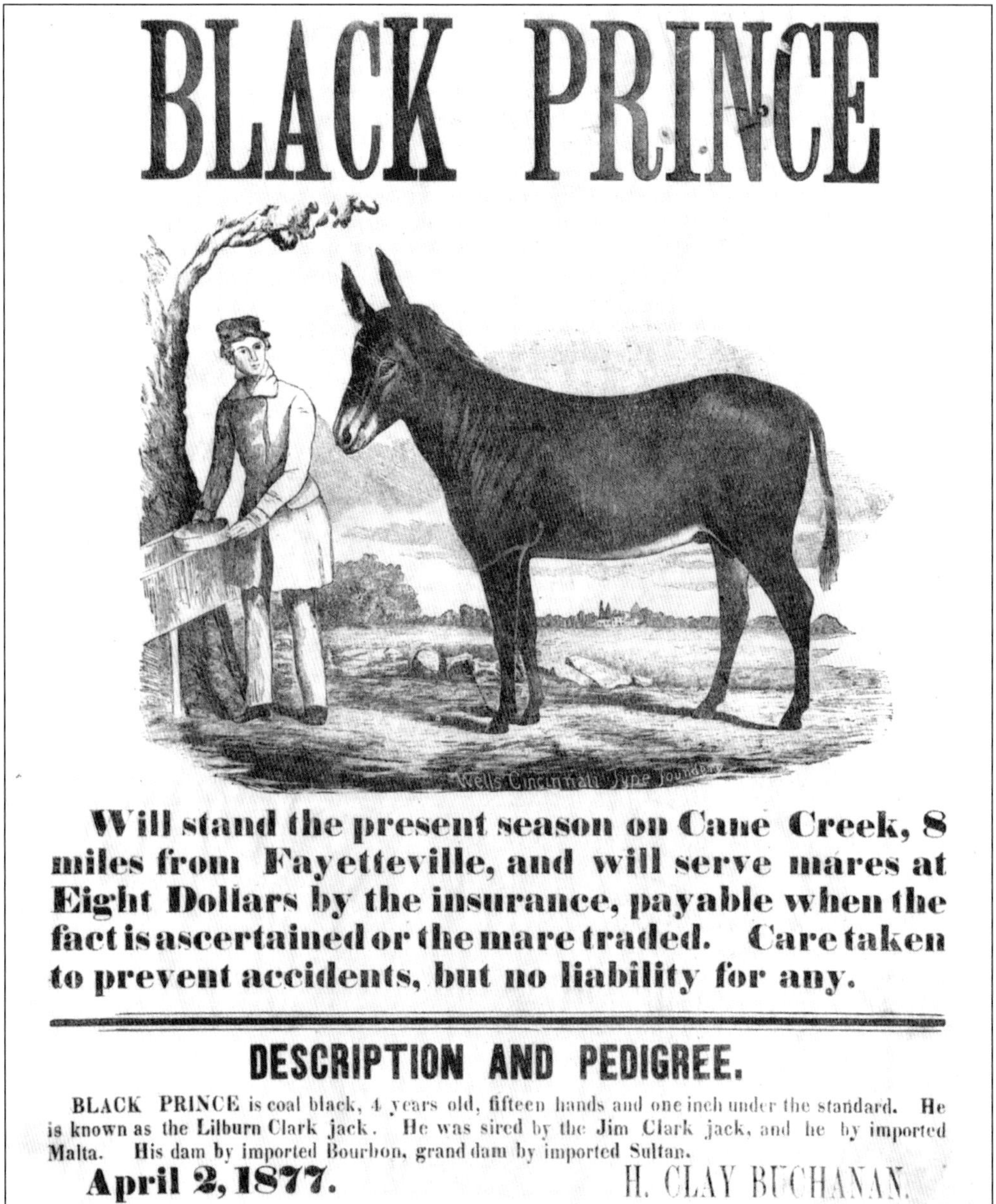
BLACK PRINCE
Wells Cincinnati Type Foundry
Will stand the present season on Cane Creek, 8 miles from Fayetteville, and will serve mares at Eight Dollars by the insurance, payable when the fact is ascertained or the mare traded. Care taken to prevent accidents, but no liability for any.
DESCRIPTION AND PEDIGREE.
BLACK PRINCE is coal black, 4 years old, fifteen hands and one inch under the standard. He is known as the Lilburn Clark jack. He was sired by the Jim Clark jack, and he by imported Malta. His dam by imported Bourbon, grand dam by imported Sultan.
April 2, 1877.
H. CLAY BUCHANAN.
Printed at the Observer Office, Fayetteville, Tenn.

This 1877 broadside advertises the jack (male donkey) Black Prince. Jack owners had two potential markets: other donkey owners and horse owners. An individual who wanted to enter the breeding business might breed his jennets (female donkeys) to Black Prince until he produced a jack of enough size for breeding to mares. A mare owner may have bred to Black Prince in order to build his herd of livestock or to enter the mule market. The American Mammoth Jack is a distinct breed and has had a registry since the 1820s. It is characterized by its height (at least 14.2 hands tall at the withers, the same minimum height requirement for a horse rather than a pony), large body, and thick bones. Pres. George Washington, at his Mount Vernon estate in Virginia, was one of the first Americans to begin breeding large jacks. (Courtesy of TSLA.)

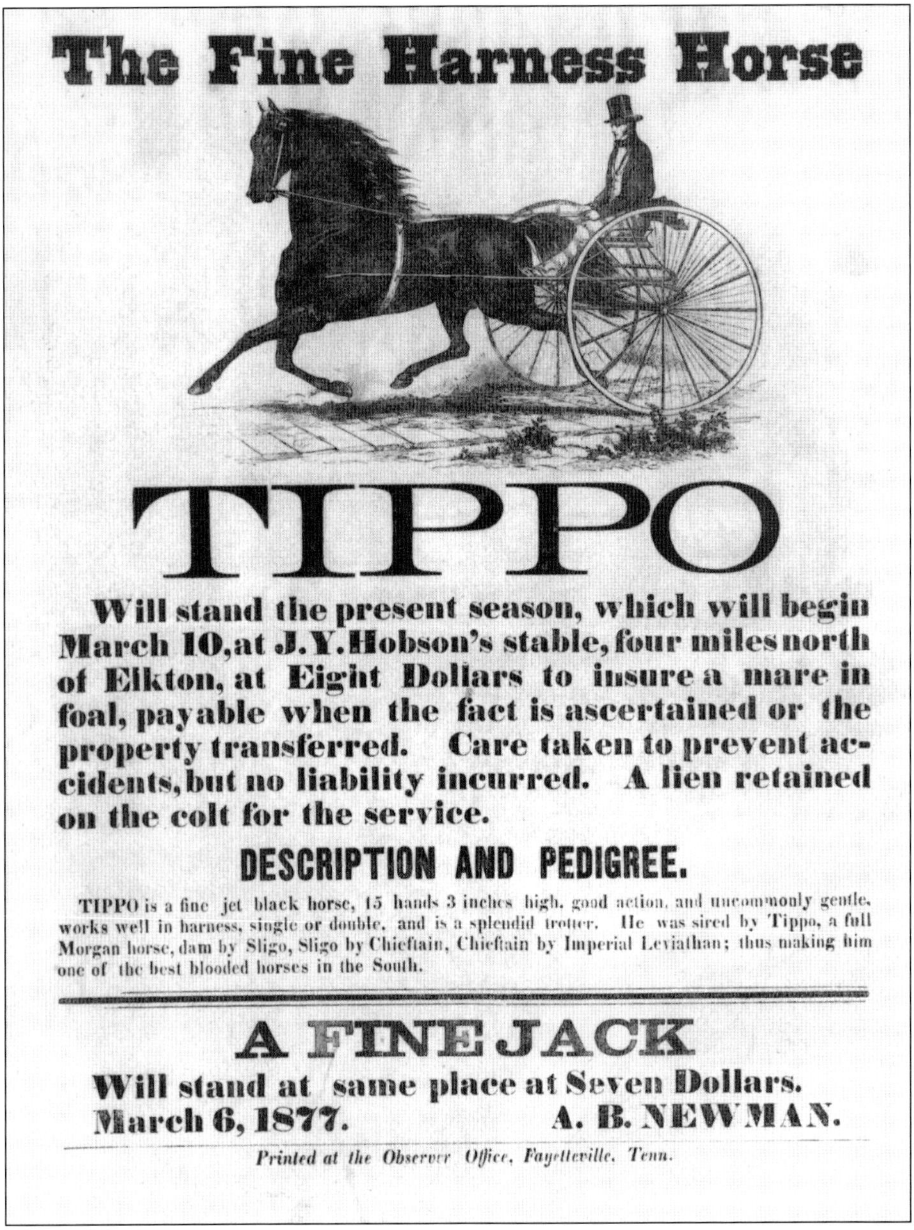

The Fine Harness Horse

TIPPO

Will stand the present season, which will begin March 10, at J. Y. Hobson's stable, four miles north of Elkton, at Eight Dollars to insure a mare in foal, payable when the fact is ascertained or the property transferred. Care taken to prevent accidents, but no liability incurred. A lien retained on the colt for the service.

DESCRIPTION AND PEDIGREE.

TIPPO is a fine jet black horse, 15 hands 3 inches high, good action, and uncommonly gentle, works well in harness, single or double, and is a splendid trotter. He was sired by Tippo, a full Morgan horse, dam by Sligo, Sligo by Chieftain, Chieftain by Imperial Leviathan; thus making him one of the best blooded horses in the South.

A FINE JACK

Will stand at same place at Seven Dollars.
March 6, 1877. A. B. NEWMAN.

Printed at the Observer Office, Fayetteville, Tenn.

This breeder has taken advantage of the opportunity to advertise both his stallion Tippo and his unnamed jack. Mules cannot reproduce, so there was always a need for quality jacks for future breeding. Because the cost of breeding a mule was quite low, many Middle Tennessean farmers raised a mule or two each year. Since most mares are able to work at a normal rate throughout most of the gestation period, breeding would not limit the horse's productivity. Once the mare foaled, farmers often let the mule colt or filly follow alongside its mother in the field. By the time the mule was ready for training, it would be used to the normal sights and sounds of farm work. After early training, mules are capable of much harder work at a younger age than horses are; farmers could sell the mules singularly or in a pair to earn extra money. Well-trained mule teams brought the highest prices at the local street markets, which were often held around the courthouse square. (Courtesy of TSLA.)

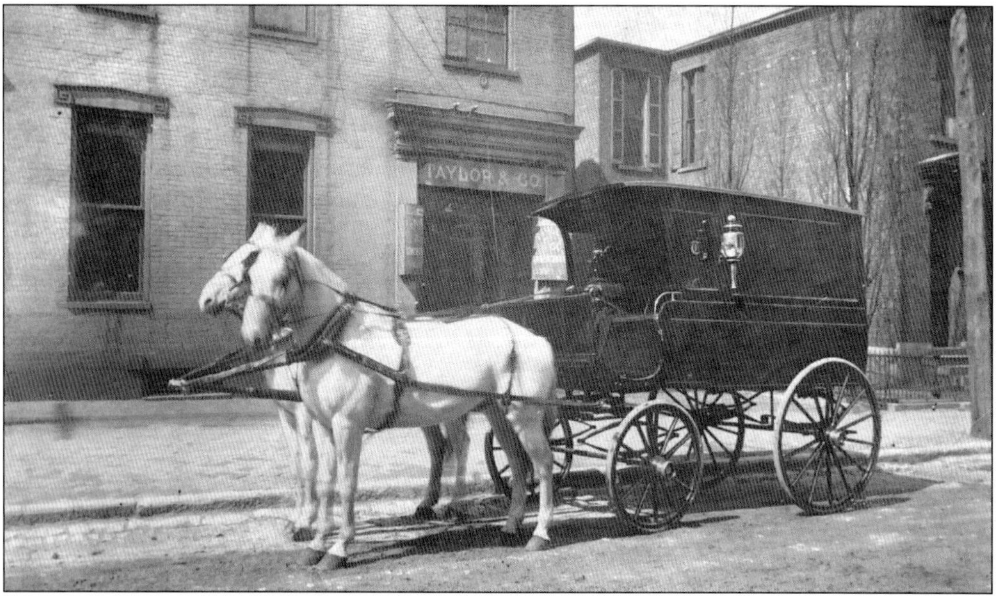

This horse-drawn hearse was just one of the seven carriages and hearses owned by Taylor and Company in Nashville. The company was established in 1888 by the Reverend Preston Taylor, who was a pastor of the Church of Disciples, a former Louisville and Chattanooga Railroad porter, and an independent contractor for the Big Sandy Railroad. Taylor and Company Funeral Directors became the largest African American undertaking business in late-19th-century Nashville. (Courtesy of TSLA.)

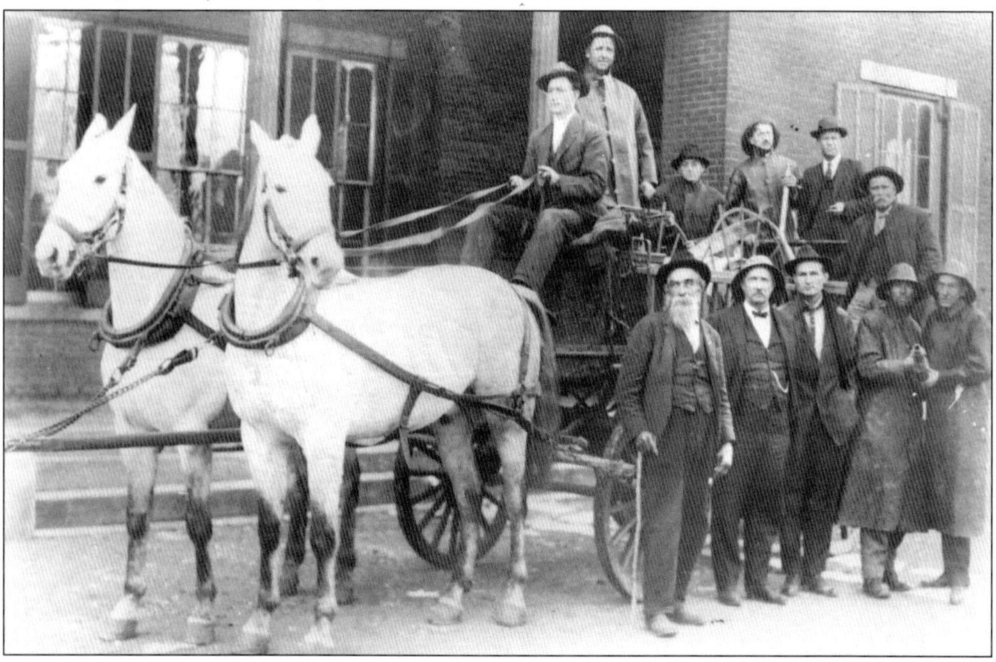

The Gallatin fire brigade used this horse-drawn wagon in 1911. Fire companies were first formed in the United States during the Colonial period, and they initially used man-drawn pumpers and hose wagons. As city streets improved and the equipment became heavier, fire brigades turned to horses to pull their equipment. (Courtesy of TSLA.)

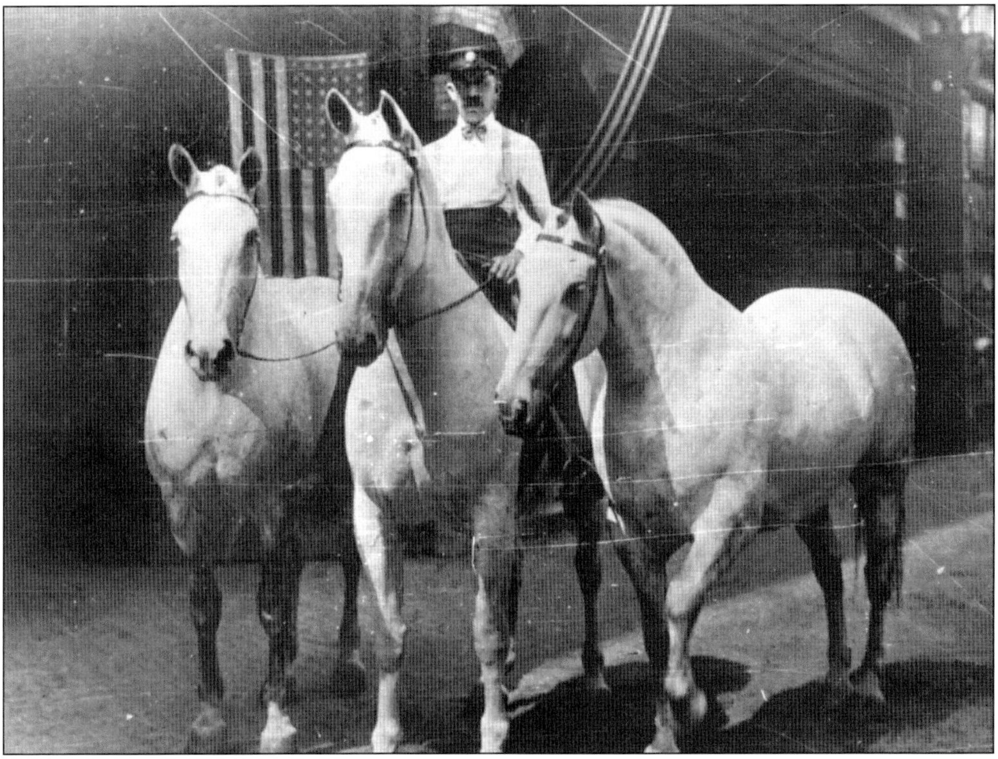

The Nashville Hook and Ladder Company No. 1 is seen above in the late 1800s showing off its three well-groomed horses. The first Nashville volunteer firefighters group formed in 1807. The city created its first paid department July 29, 1860, and the chief, J. S. Dashiell, quickly purchased three horse-drawn steam engines. Nashville's Engine No. 6 horses, seen below, are illustrative of the large and well-muscled 1890s fire company horses. Fire stations included stabling areas for all of the horses, and the harnesses were often stored suspended above the entrance to enable quick hitching once the alarm was sounded. These Nashville horses may have represented Middle Tennessee in national competitions, which pitted fire brigades against one another and the clock to demonstrate their ability to arrive at a fire in record time. (Courtesy of TSLA.)

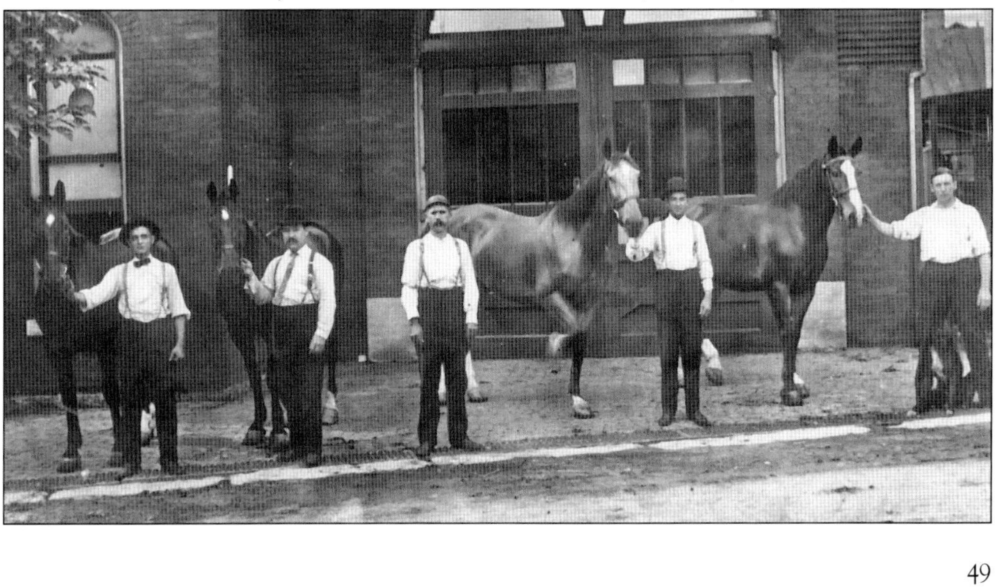

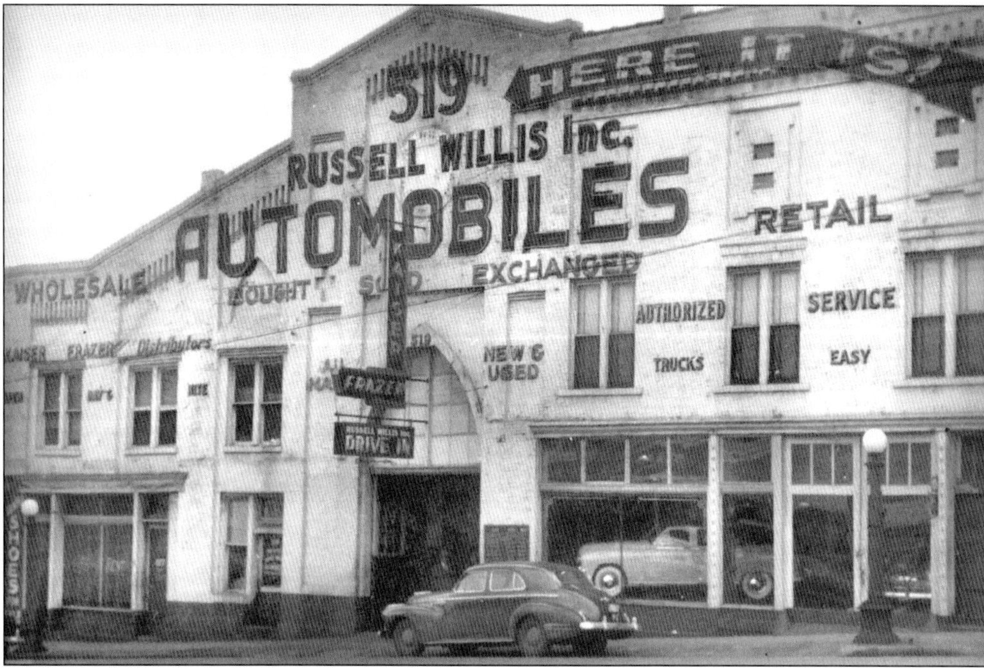

The Waldorf Stable on Nashville's Broadway Avenue symbolizes Middle Tennessee's urban horses of the late 19th and early 20th centuries. This building was subsequently transformed into a car dealership—a logical transition. Large businesses, such as breweries or packinghouses, used horses to transport their materials and finished products. (Courtesy of Gore Center.)

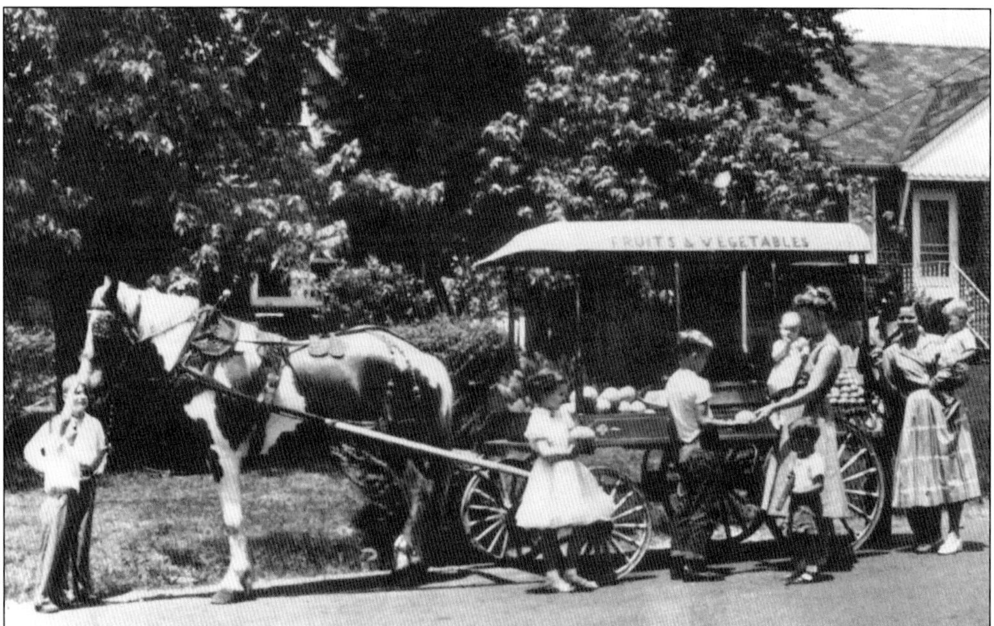

This horse-drawn produce cart traveled the streets of Nashville in the 1930s. Before World War II, it was not uncommon to see one-horse carts or wagons in both small and large urban areas. Farmers from the surrounding area brought each day's harvest to the central market to sell from their wagons. (Courtesy of TSLA.)

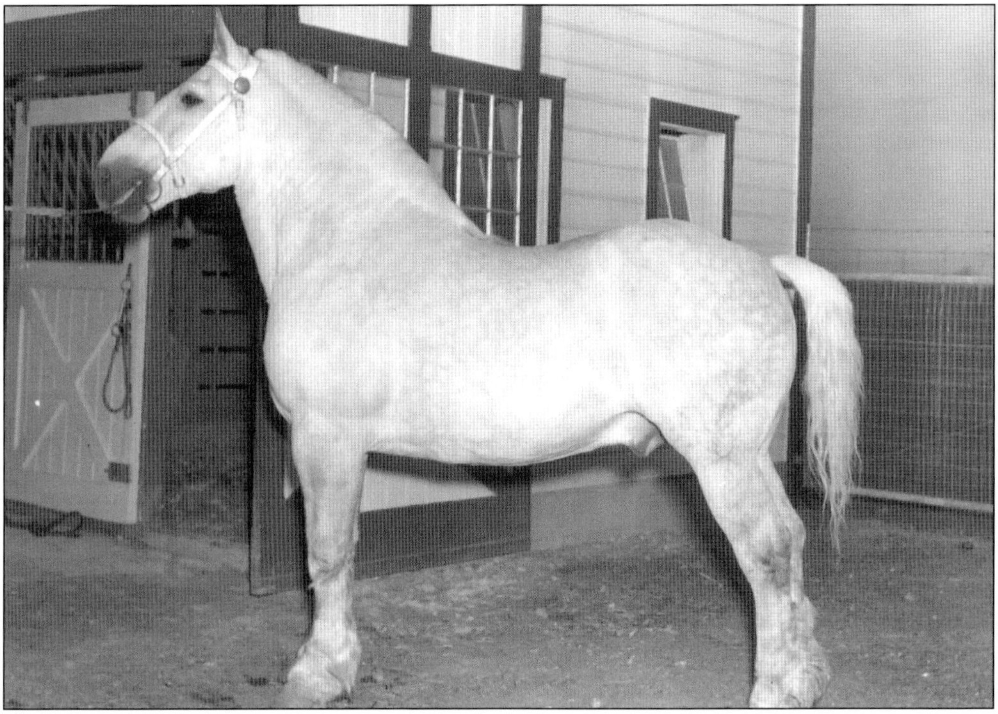

This Percheron stallion stood at Harwick Farms in Cleveland, Tennessee, during the 1920s. Although European draft horses were not uncommon in Middle Tennessee, the region did not breed large numbers of Percherons, Belgians, Clydesdales, or Shires like the upper Midwest did. Despite their relatively small numbers, draft horses were bred with the same dedication and skill as were the more popular Middle Tennessee horses. (Courtesy of TSLA.)

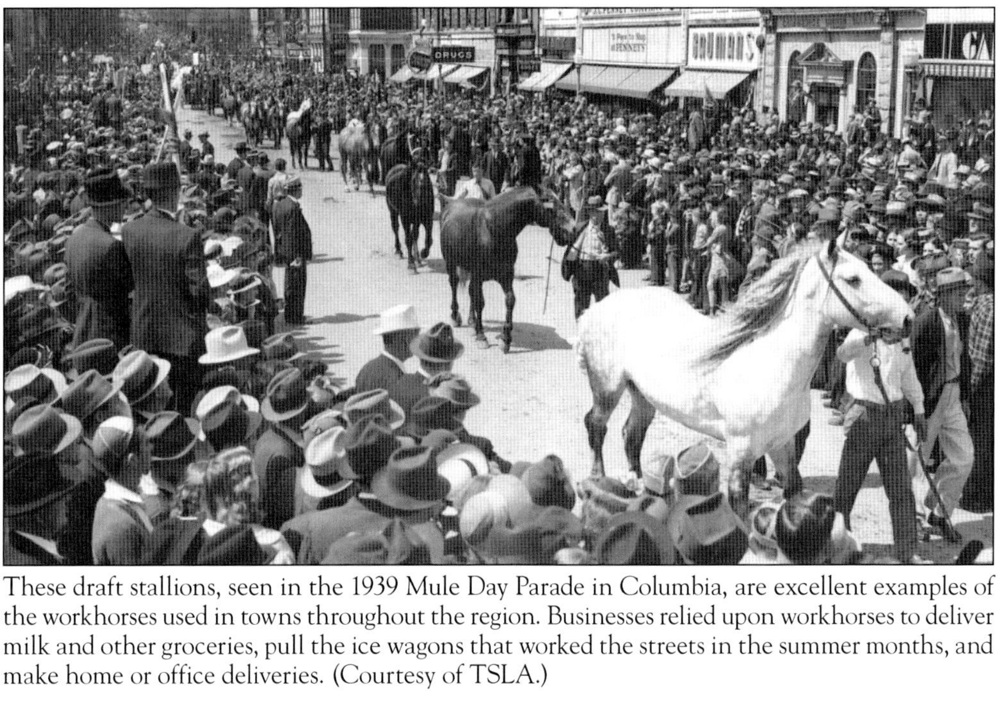

These draft stallions, seen in the 1939 Mule Day Parade in Columbia, are excellent examples of the workhorses used in towns throughout the region. Businesses relied upon workhorses to deliver milk and other groceries, pull the ice wagons that worked the streets in the summer months, and make home or office deliveries. (Courtesy of TSLA.)

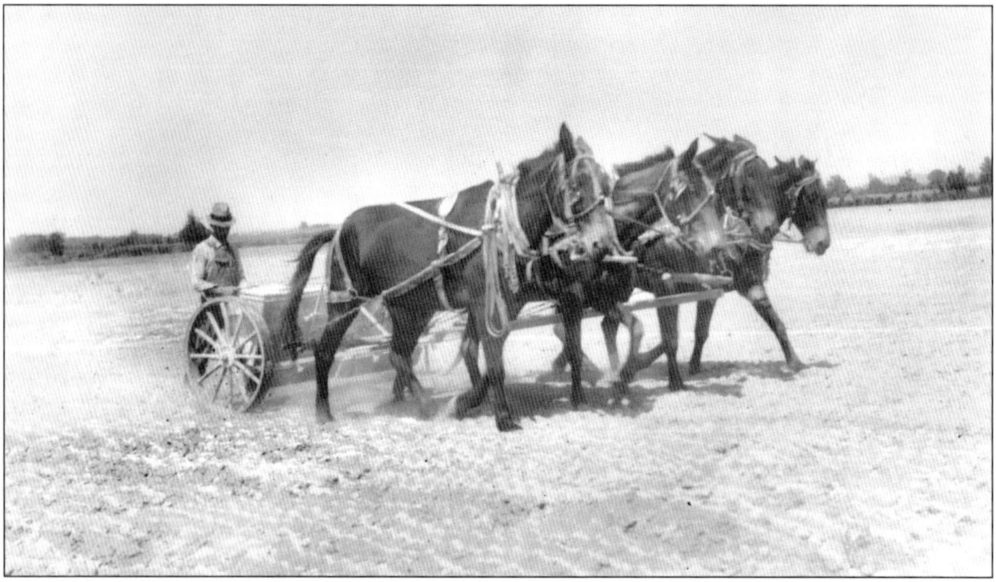

This four-mule team working a Middle Tennessee field in the 1930s is symbolic of the region and the time period. After several months of training, the mules learned to move as a team, keeping a steady pace that allowed them to work from sunrise to sunset. During the Depression, mules were an important resource for families without the cash to buy gasoline or tractor parts. (Courtesy of TSLA.)

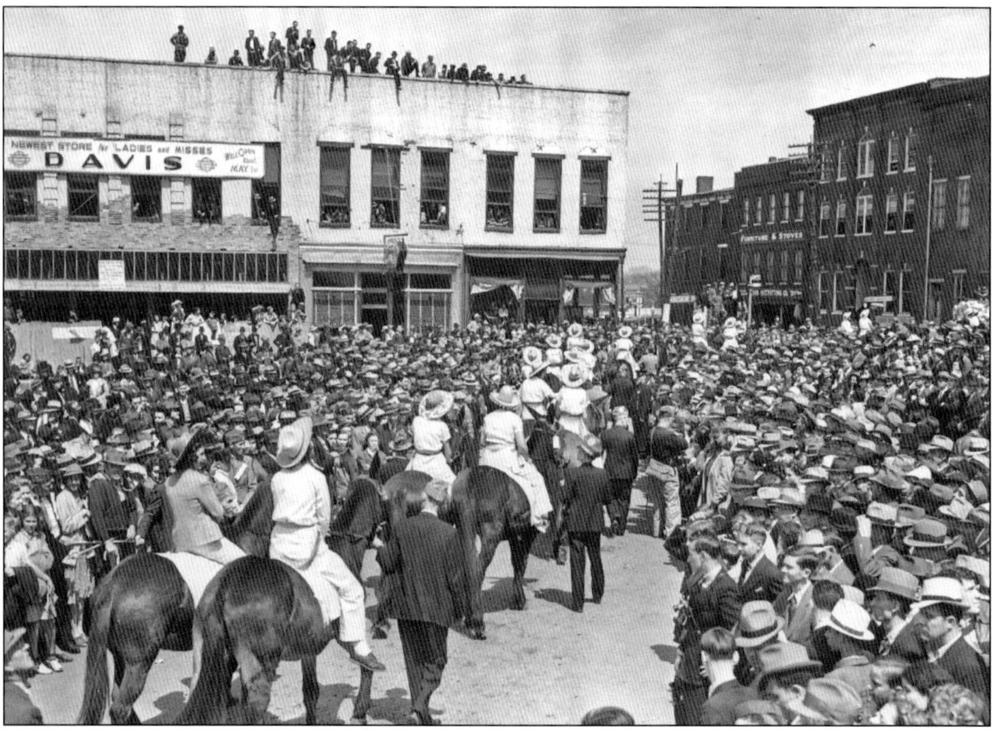

The Mule Day Parade in Columbia has been an important Middle Tennessee event since its inception in 1934. The parade grew out of the older Columbia Mule Day (held on the first Monday in April since 1840) as part of the larger Breeder's and Livestock Show. (Courtesy of TSLA.)

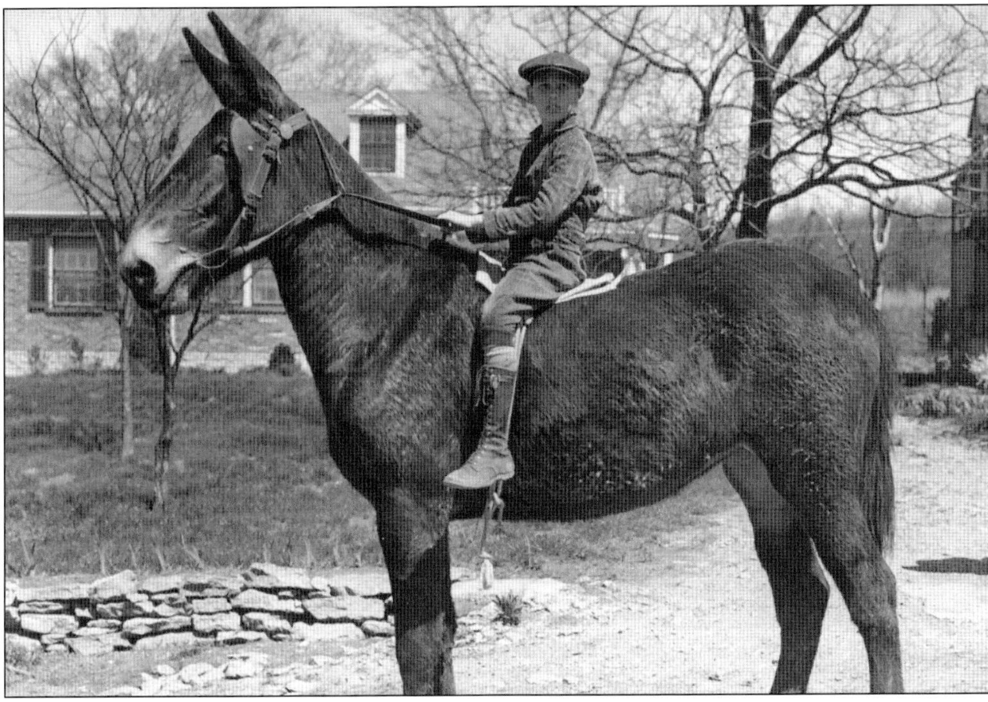

This farm boy, J. B. Napier of Columbia, rides his family's 18-hand-tall mule in the 1939 Mule Day Parade. This mule was reportedly the largest in that year's parade. Mule owners used the parade as an opportunity to show off their mules or to sell their stock. (Courtesy of TSLA.)

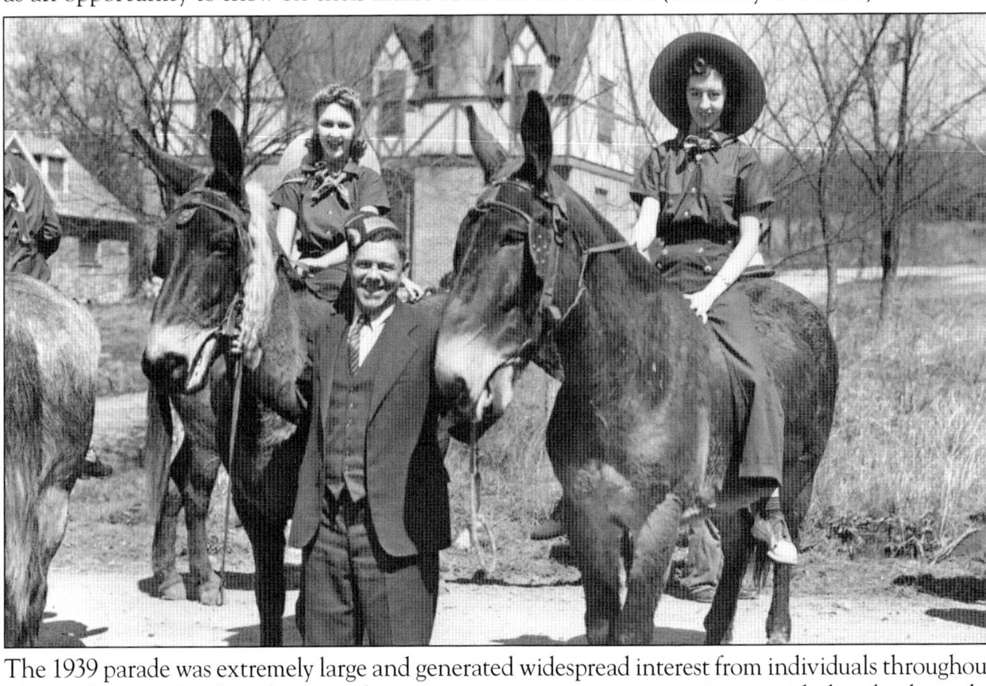

The 1939 parade was extremely large and generated widespread interest from individuals throughout Maury County. In this photograph, two young women are preparing to ride bareback in the parade. Although other Middle Tennessee towns had mule sale days and parades, none of them have ever reached the size of Columbia's. (Courtesy of TSLA.)

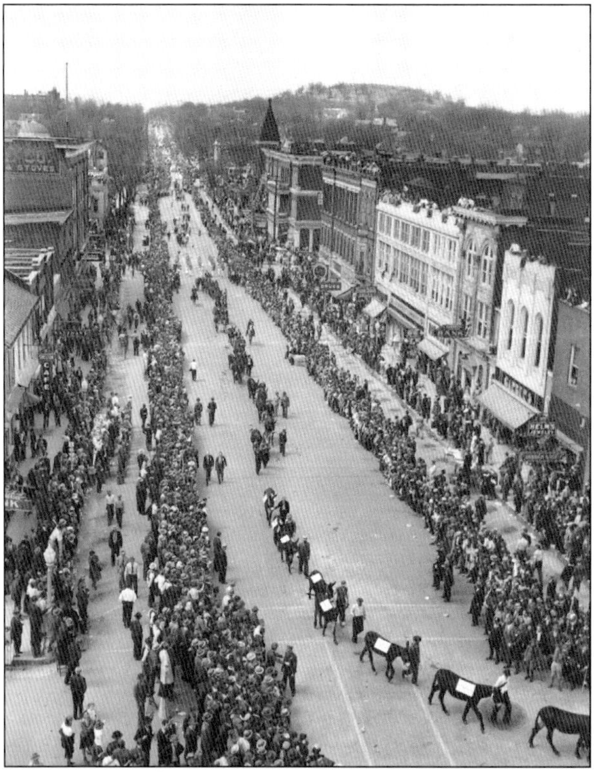

This long view of the 1940 Columbia Mule Day Parade shows the large number of spectators and participants. The 1940 parade marked the centennial of Columbia's mule day and included a 2-mile-long procession of mules, horses, and Middle Tennesseans. This photograph reemphasizes the importance of the horse and mule in Middle Tennessee. (Courtesy of TSLA.)

The 1940 Columbia Mule Day Parade was one of the largest of its kind in the world and attracted national-level visitors. In this photograph, Tennessee's governor, Prentice Cooper (center), escorts the Democratic Party's national chairman, James A. Farley (right). The mule day visitors might have been well known for their politics, but the mule was the day's true celebrity. (Courtesy of TSLA.)

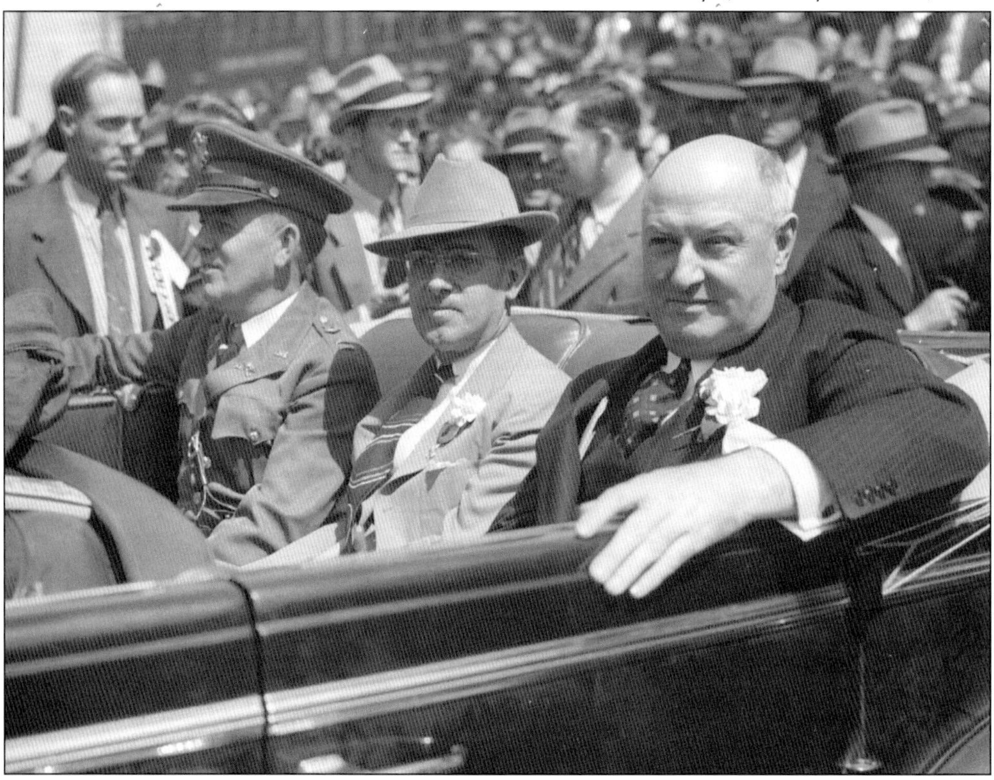

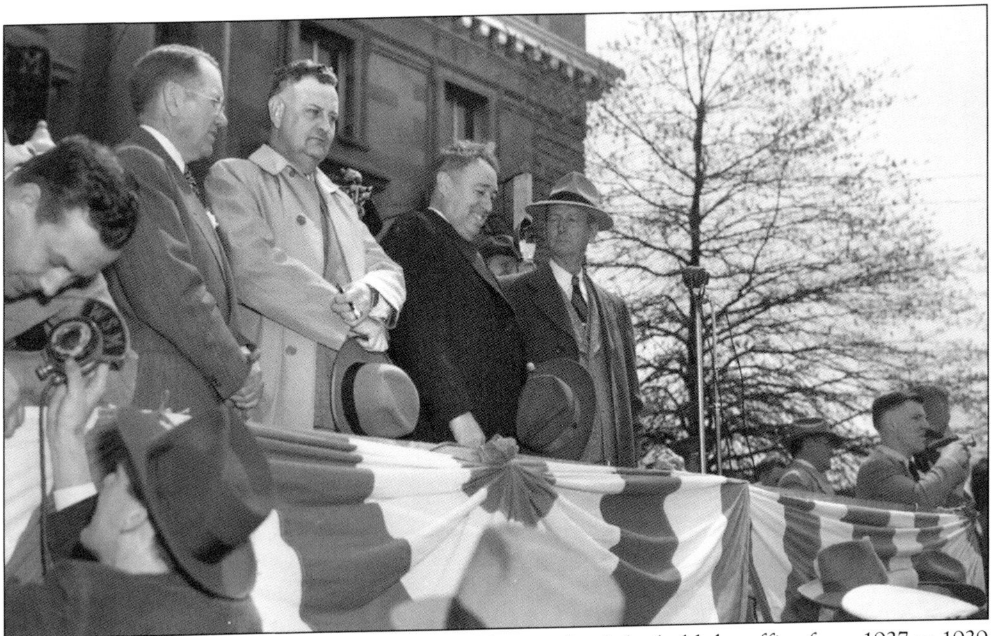

Tennessee governor Gordon Browning, second from right, (who held the office from 1937 to 1939 and from 1949 to 1953) and Gen. Jonathan M. Wainwright IV of the U.S. Army (standing far right) watch as the 1949 Columbia Mule Day Parade passes by. The Mule Day festivities dwindled after 1950. In 1974, the Maury County Bridle and Saddle Club reorganized Mule Day, and the parade has flourished ever since. (Courtesy of TSLA.)

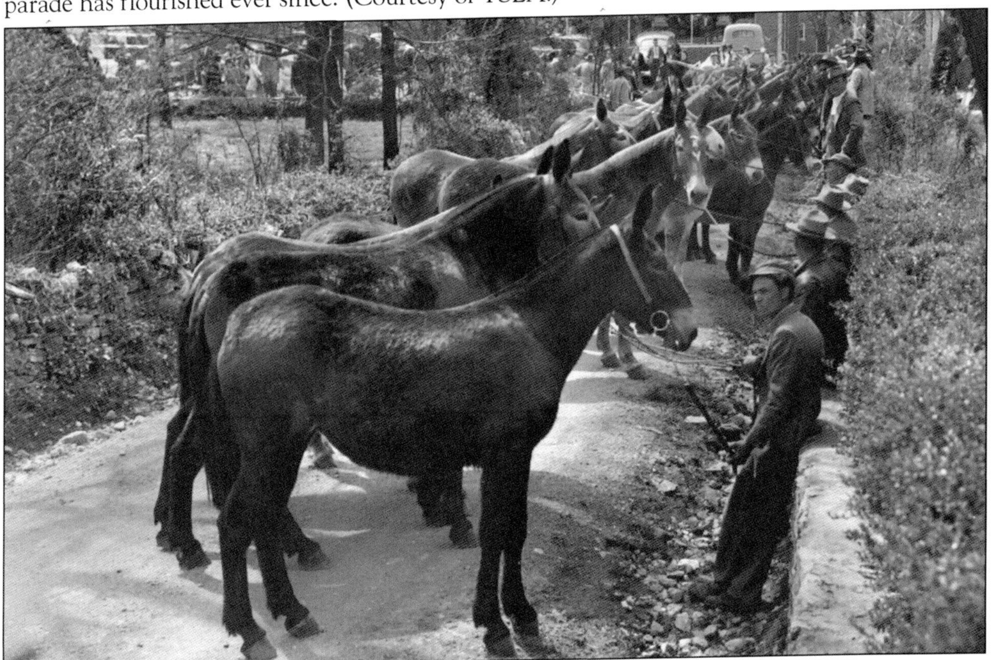

These mules are standing on a Columbia side street waiting for the 1949 parade to begin—and, perhaps, for potential buyers to take notice. Mule breeding in Middle Tennessee reached an all-time low from the 1960s to the 1980s, but in the last decade, mule breeders have seen a marked increase in demand. (Courtesy of TSLA.)

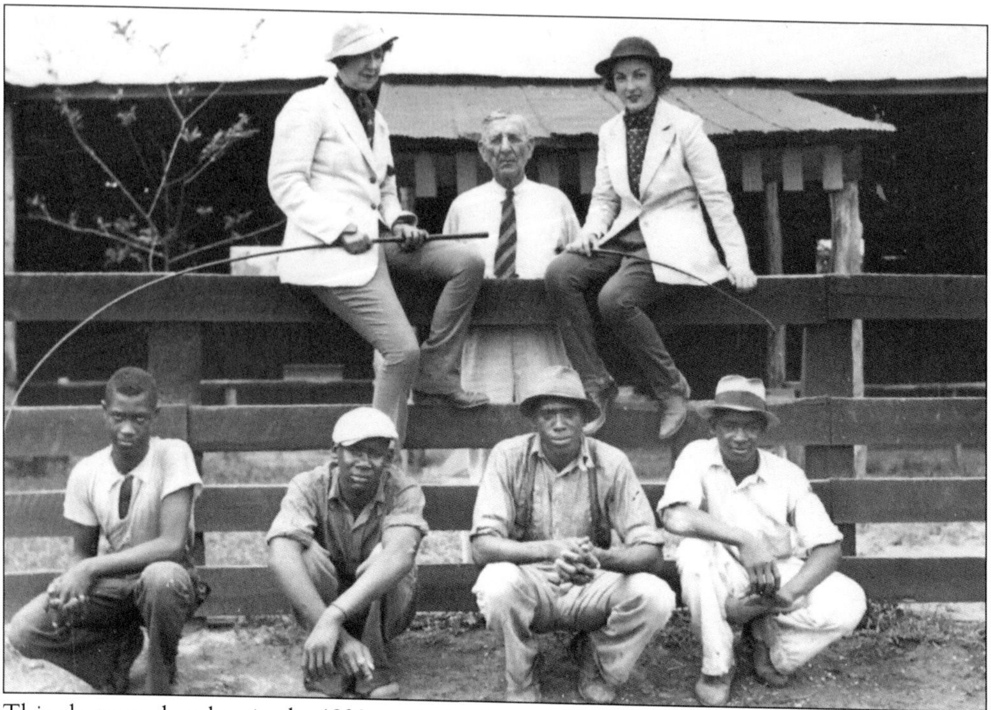

This photograph, taken in the 1930s at Dude Camp Stables in Estill Springs, symbolizes another type of workhorse: the lesson horse. Most training and breeding stables that taught riding had a group of horses for lessons. Pictured are Mary Giltner Crawford (back left); her father, Dr. G. B. Giltner (center); and her assistants and grooms. (Courtesy of Gore Center.)

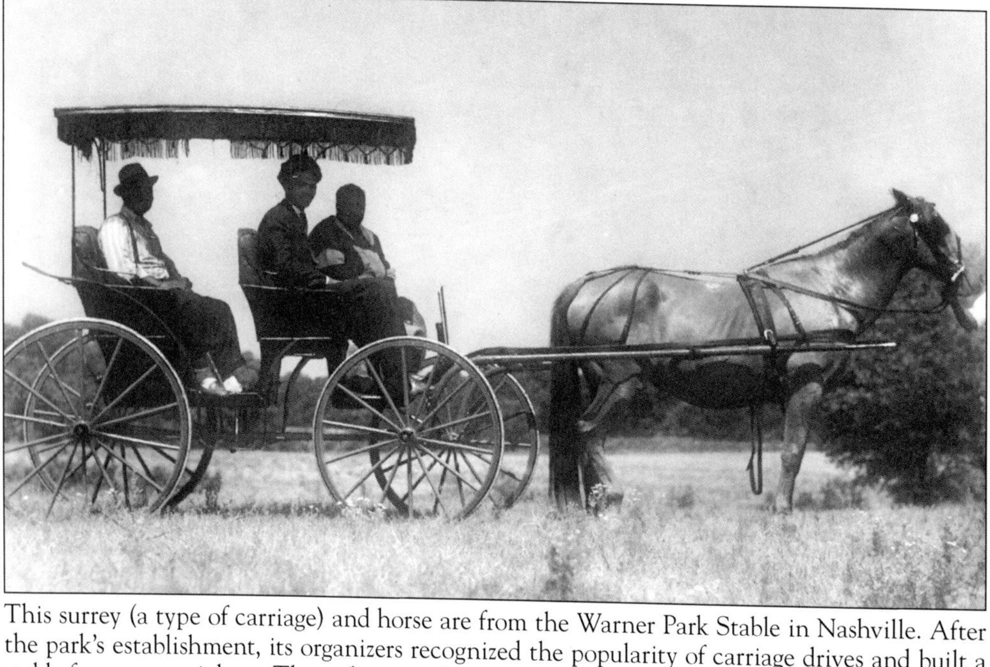

This surrey (a type of carriage) and horse are from the Warner Park Stable in Nashville. After the park's establishment, its organizers recognized the popularity of carriage drives and built a stable for commercial use. These three unidentified African Americans, seen here in 1940, most likely rented this surrey and horse for the day. (Courtesy of Gore Center.)

Four

Tennessee Walking Horses

After the decline of influential 19th-century Thoroughbred and Standardbred breeders, other Middle Tennesseans began to have wide success with the popular Tennessee Walking Horse. Bred as a strong work horse that was also comfortable for riding, the Tennessee Walker was the first horse breed named after a state. Breeding gaited horses, such as Saddlebreds and Morgans, with Standardbreds and Thoroughbreds created a horse known for its stamina and smooth yet showy motion. The establishment of an official breeding registry in 1935 helped solidify the breed's identity and provided direction for future crosses. In the 1930s, Walking Horses filled local shows' pleasure classes, and they made up a large percentage of the mounts for popular group trail rides. Henry Davis's establishment of the Tennessee Walking Horse National Celebration in 1939 resulted in a competition that now regularly draws over 2,000 horses to Shelbyville for the 11 days prior to Labor Day.

Because the Walking Horse is a regional native, the number of breeding farms and training stables in Middle Tennessee has always been high, especially in Bedford, Cannon, Coffee, Maury, Marshall, and Rutherford Counties. Some of the first breeders and trainers of Tennessee Walkers to emerge after the breed's foundation lines were established included Doug Stubblefield, Gene Paul Mayfield, Fred Kirby, C. A. Bobo, Garland Bradshaw, Sam Paschal, Joe F. Rankin, S. W. and Steve Beech, and Mary Ann Gray, the first woman to be a noted professional trainer in the Walking Horse industry. By the 1970s, the second generation of trainers and breeders began to establish stables beyond Middle Tennessee, earning national recognition. This chapter will concentrate on the 1930s and 1940s, pivotal years in the popularization and breeding of the Tennessee Walking Horse.

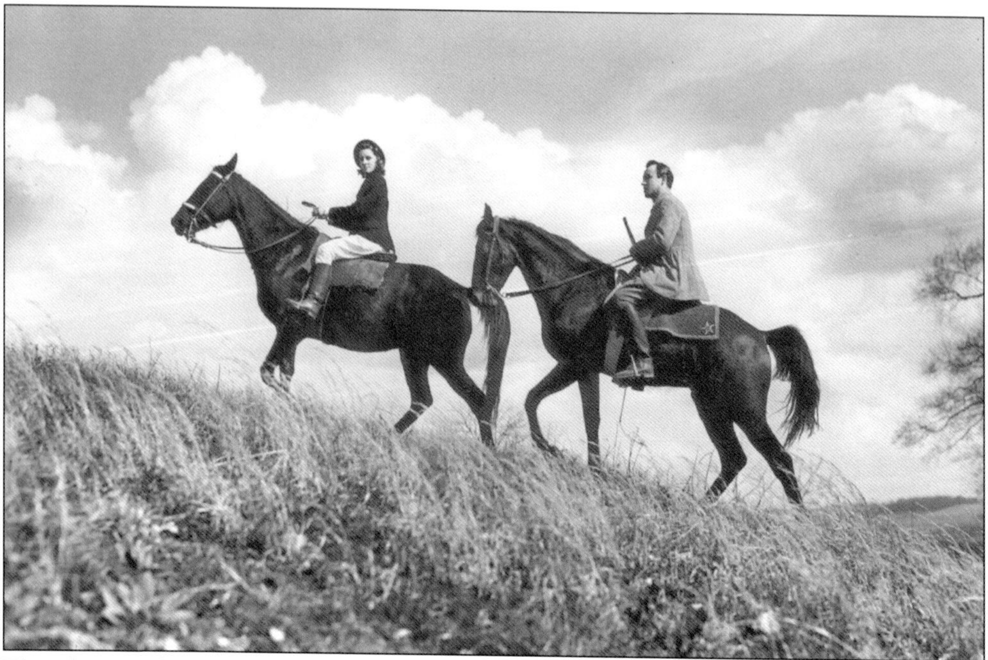

This photograph shows Mabel Blackman of Wartrace and Calvin Houghland of Nashville scaling a hill near Wartrace. This image exemplifies the emphasis placed upon horses and social recreation from the 1920s to the 1940s. It is quite likely that Blackman's horse is a Tennessee Walking Horse and that the two were part of a larger group of horses and riders. (Courtesy of TSLA.)

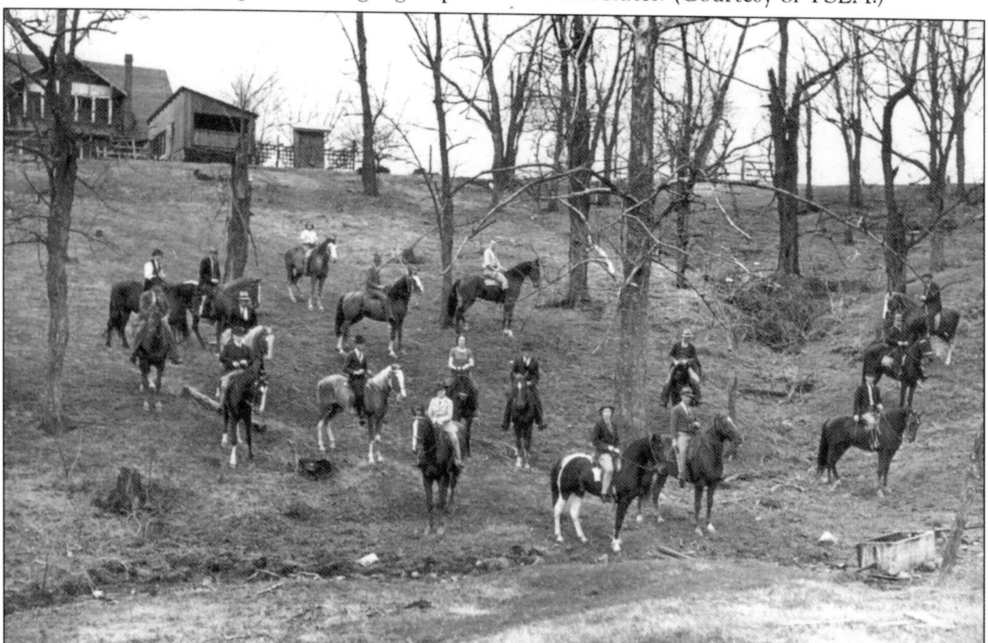

This group trail ride in March 1938 began in Wartrace. A small town in the south-central section of Middle Tennessee, Wartrace emerged as a center for Walking Horse activity. In additional to opportunities for socialization, long trail rides also allowed young horses to "gain miles," helping them become better trained and conditioned. (Courtesy of TSLA.)

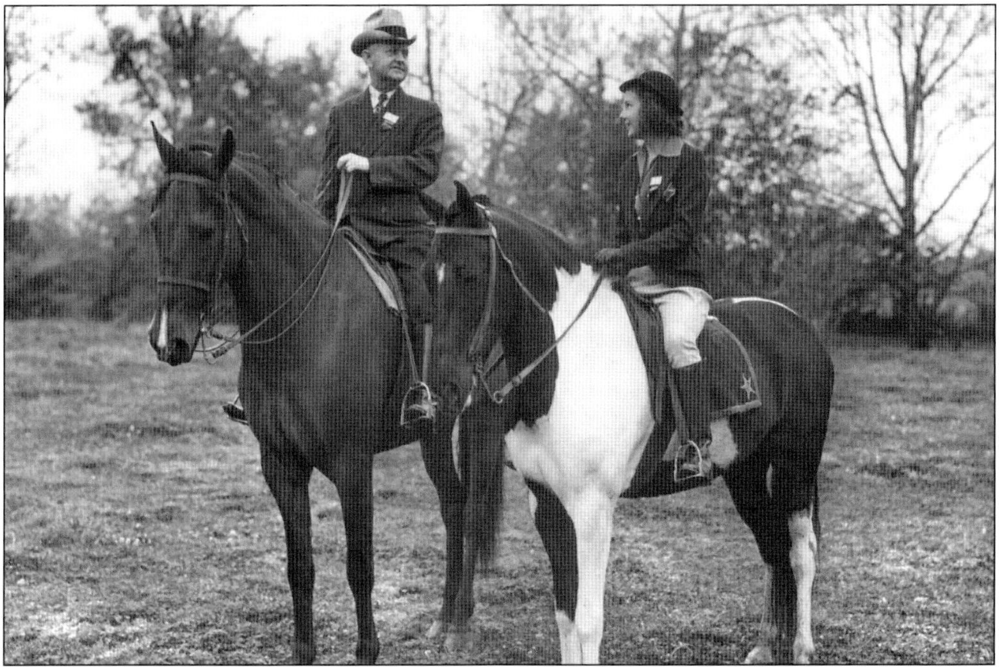

This photograph shows A. B. and Mary Womack of Murfreesboro participating in an April 1939 trail ride in Chapel Hill. The Womack family has been very involved with the Tennessee Walking Horse as breeders, and Dr. Bob Womack has written the definitive history of the breed. (Courtesy of TSLA.)

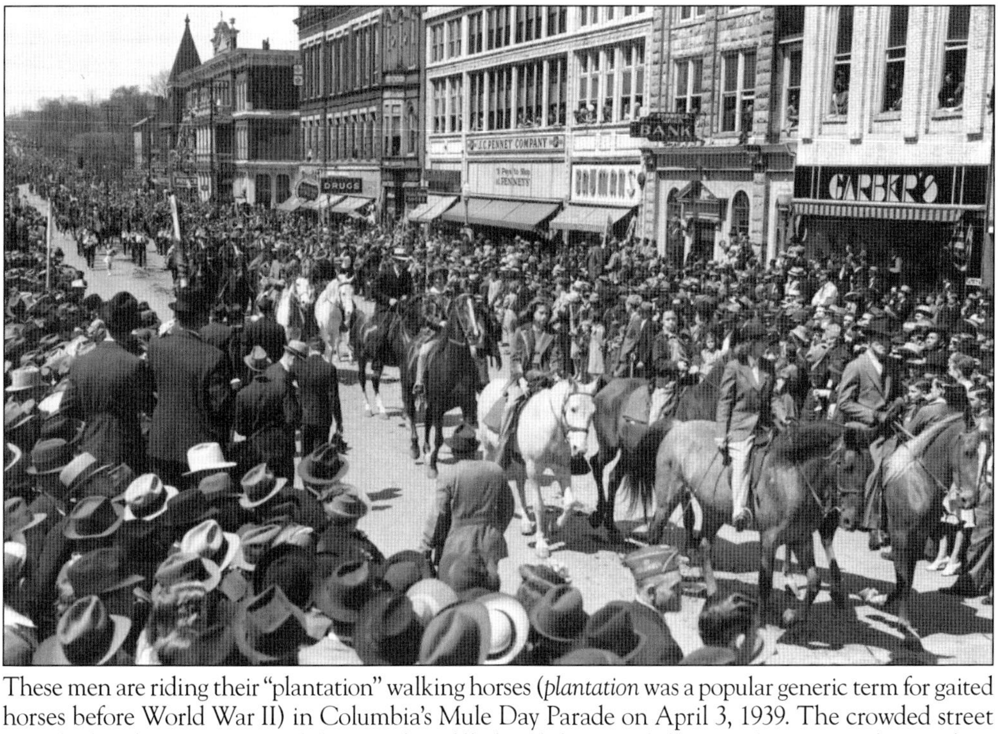

These men are riding their "plantation" walking horses (*plantation* was a popular generic term for gaited horses before World War II) in Columbia's Mule Day Parade on April 3, 1939. The crowded street is packed with spectators, and the parade is filled with horses of all types. (Courtesy of TSLA.)

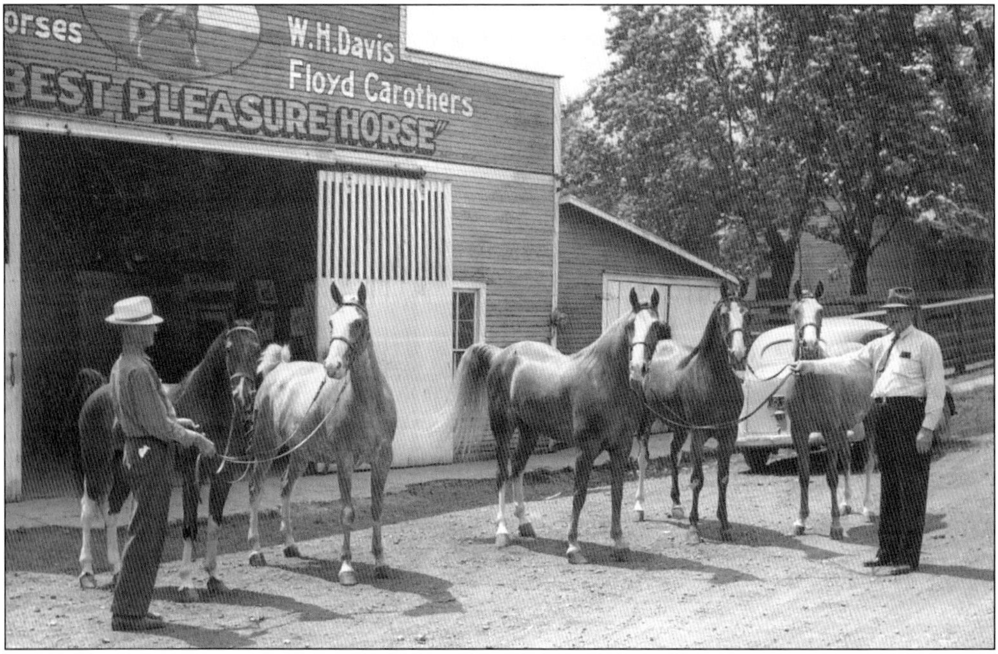

The horses shown here in June 1940 were part of the Shelbyville Ride-a-thon as it passed through Wartrace, a popular summer activity. A long-distance route was laid out ahead of time, and entrants rode individually or in groups. Horse owners not only socialized but also took the opportunity to show off their horses, especially those available for purchase. (Courtesy of TSLA.)

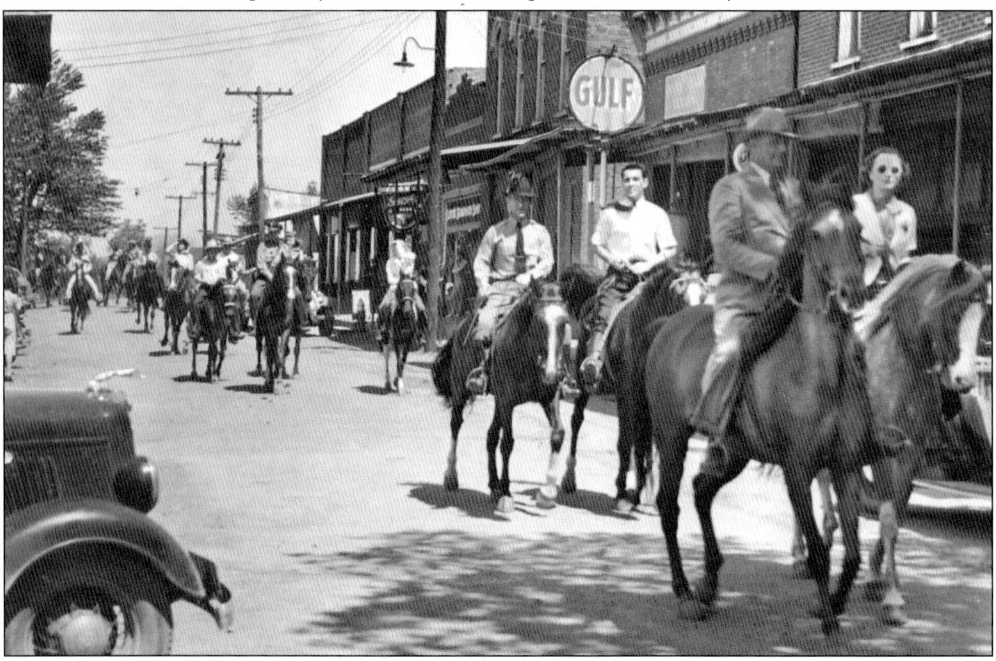

This photograph, taken in 1939 or the 1940s, shows the parade that was held in honor of the Tennessee Walking Horse National Celebration in Shelbyville. Although this image clearly shows several female parade riders, the majority of the early Tennessee Walking Horse industry professionals were men. The few women were usually wives or daughters of professionals. (Courtesy of Gore Center.)

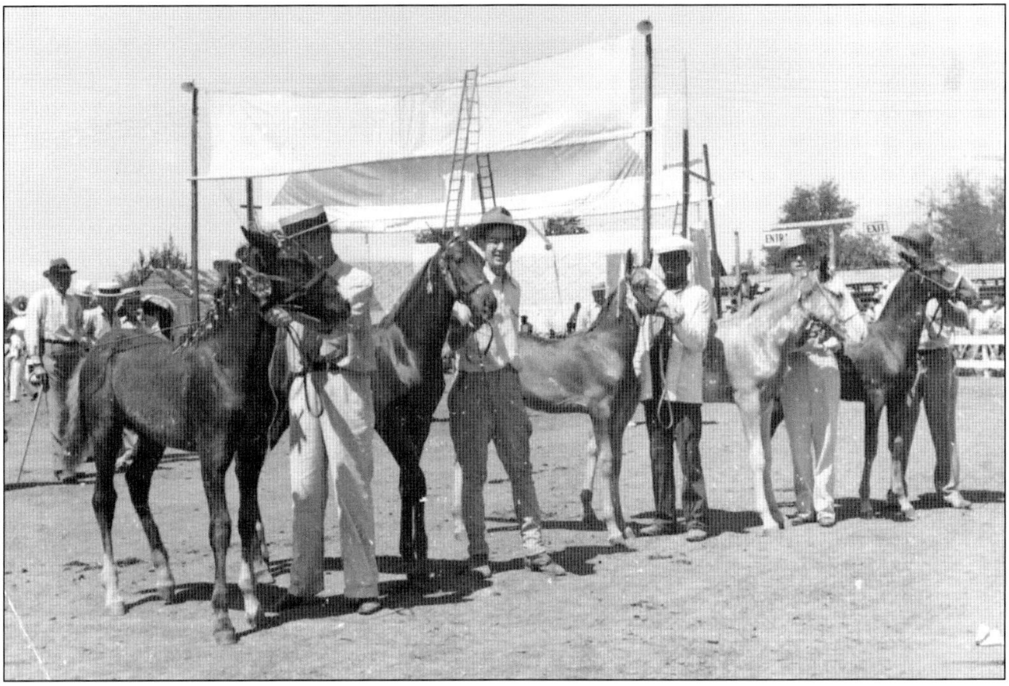

These weanlings (horses less than a year old that are no longer nursing) are competing in the Celebration's original show ring in 1939 or the 1940s. Of particular interest is the African American competitor whose entry has won a ribbon. (Courtesy of Gore Center.)

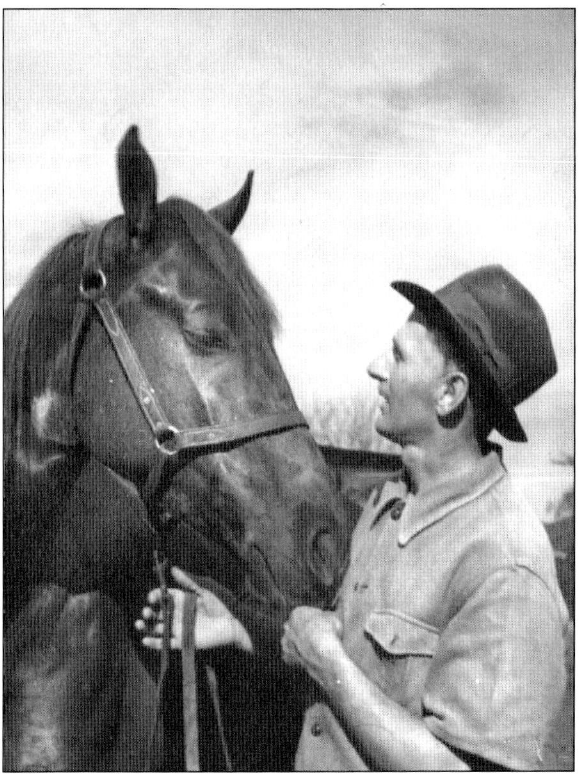

Floyd Carothers, one of the important early Walking Horse trainers, is shown here with perhaps his most famous horse, Strolling Jim 410315. This chestnut gelding became the first Grand Champion Walking Horse at the inaugural Tennessee Walking Horse National Celebration in 1939. Henry Davis and Floyd Carothers discovered him in Viola, where his breeder, Ed Gilliam, used him for working and riding. (Courtesy of Gore Center.)

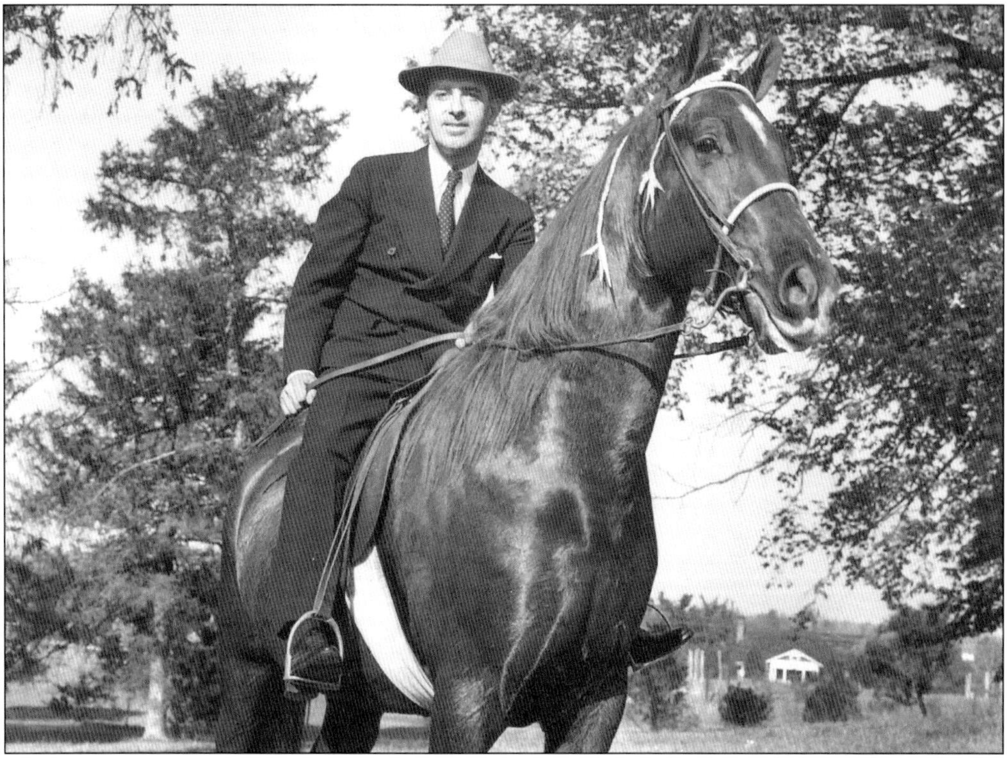

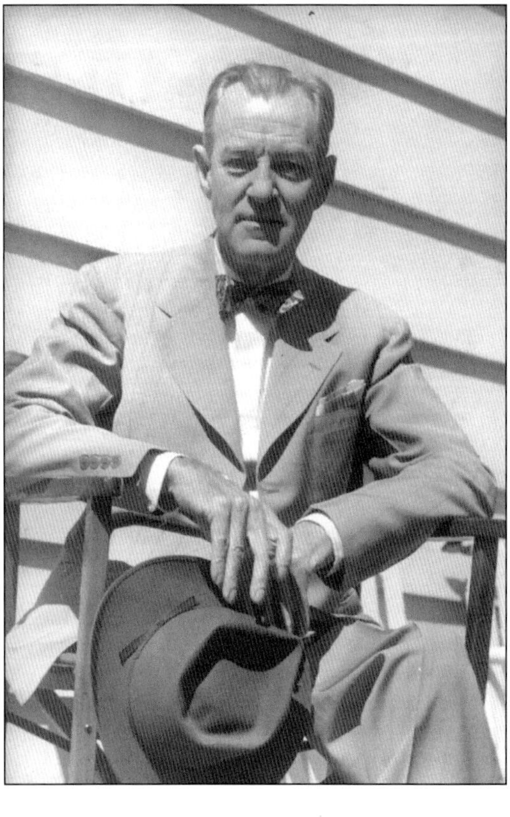

Tennessee governor Prentice Cooper (who held the office from 1939 to 1945) enjoys his ride on the 1939 Grand Champion Strolling Jim in Shelbyville. Governor Cooper, a Shelbyville native, was a strong supporter of Tennessee agriculture. The growing Walking Horse industry was an important part of the economy. (Courtesy of TSLA.)

Gilbert MacWilliams Orr, a lawyer in Maury County, was one of the earliest and most persuasive promoters of the Tennessee Walking Horse. Often called "Mr. Tennessee Walking Horse," Orr served the Walking Horse as a contributor to the Nashville newspapers and as an announcer at many of the horse shows. (Courtesy of Gore Center.)

Beyond the horse world, Lem Motlow is probably best known for his association with the Jack Daniels Distillery in Lynchburg. However, Motlow was also a horse lover, and he owned several excellent Tennessee Walking Horses. Moore County has continued to maintain its ties to the Walking Horse through the Tennessee Walking Horse Museum in Lynchburg, which is supported in part by the Jack Daniels Distillery. (Courtesy of Gore Center.)

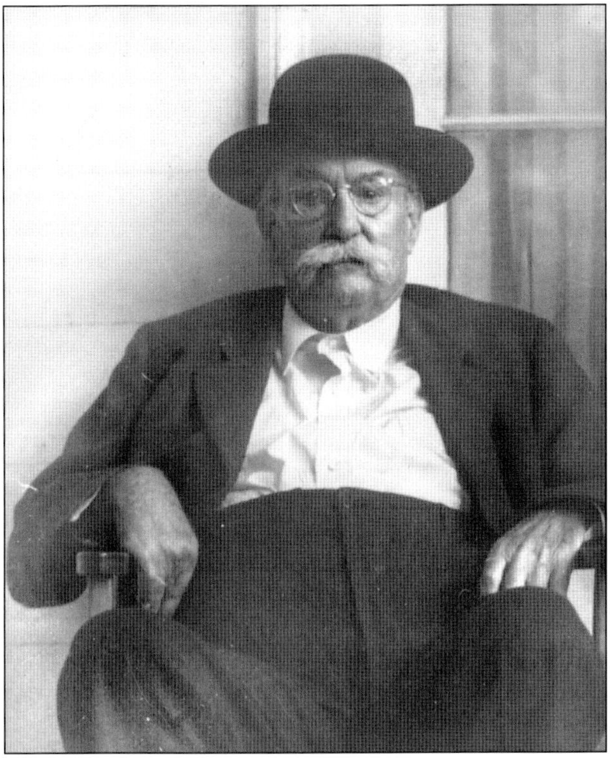

Chief's Allen was a Tennessee Walking Horse stallion owned by Lem Motlow of Lynchburg. The horse won an impressive 20 blue ribbons in the course of one show year. He went on to sire 83 foals. (Courtesy of Gore Center.)

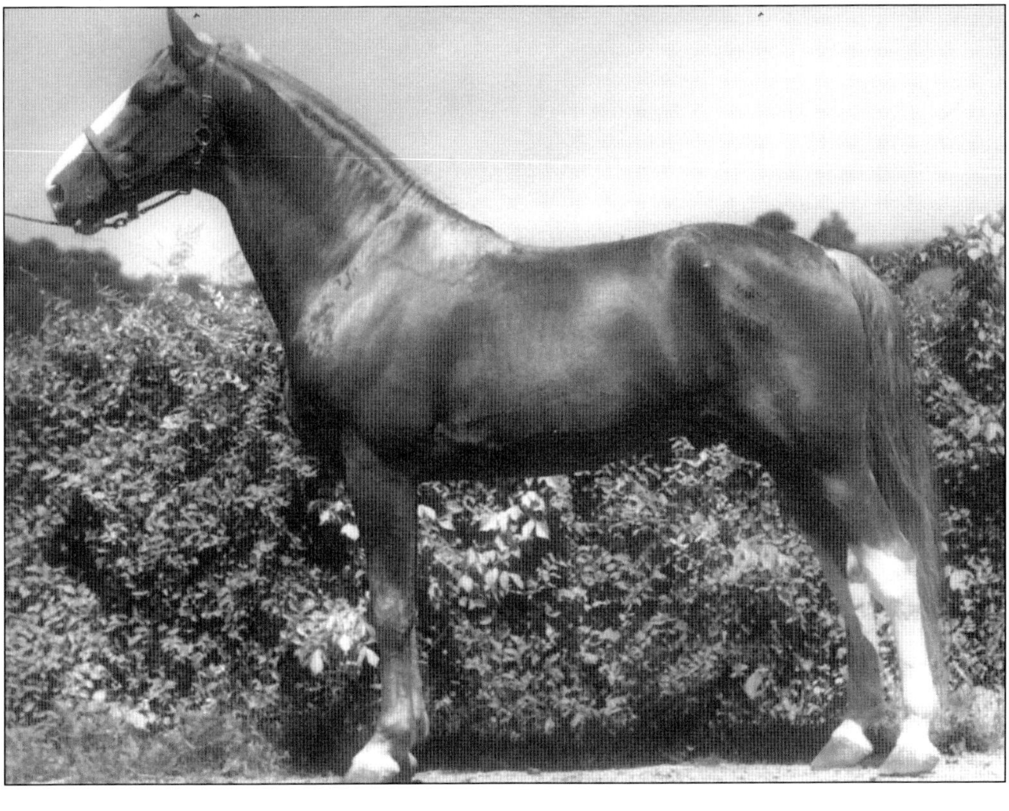

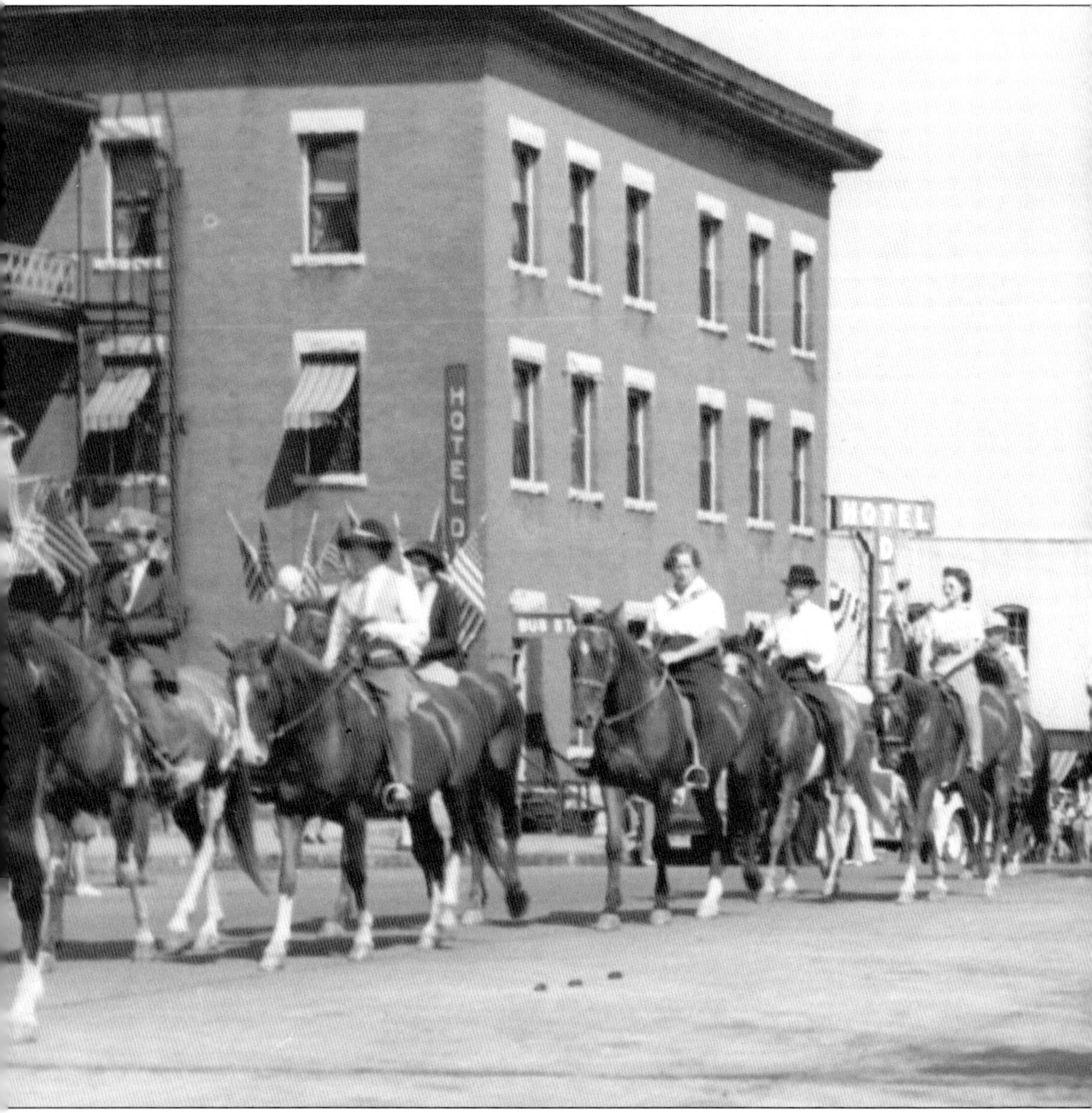

This 1939 or early-1940s photograph has captured the Tennessee Walking Horse National Celebration parade in Shelbyville as it crosses the Bedford County courthouse square. The Celebration has

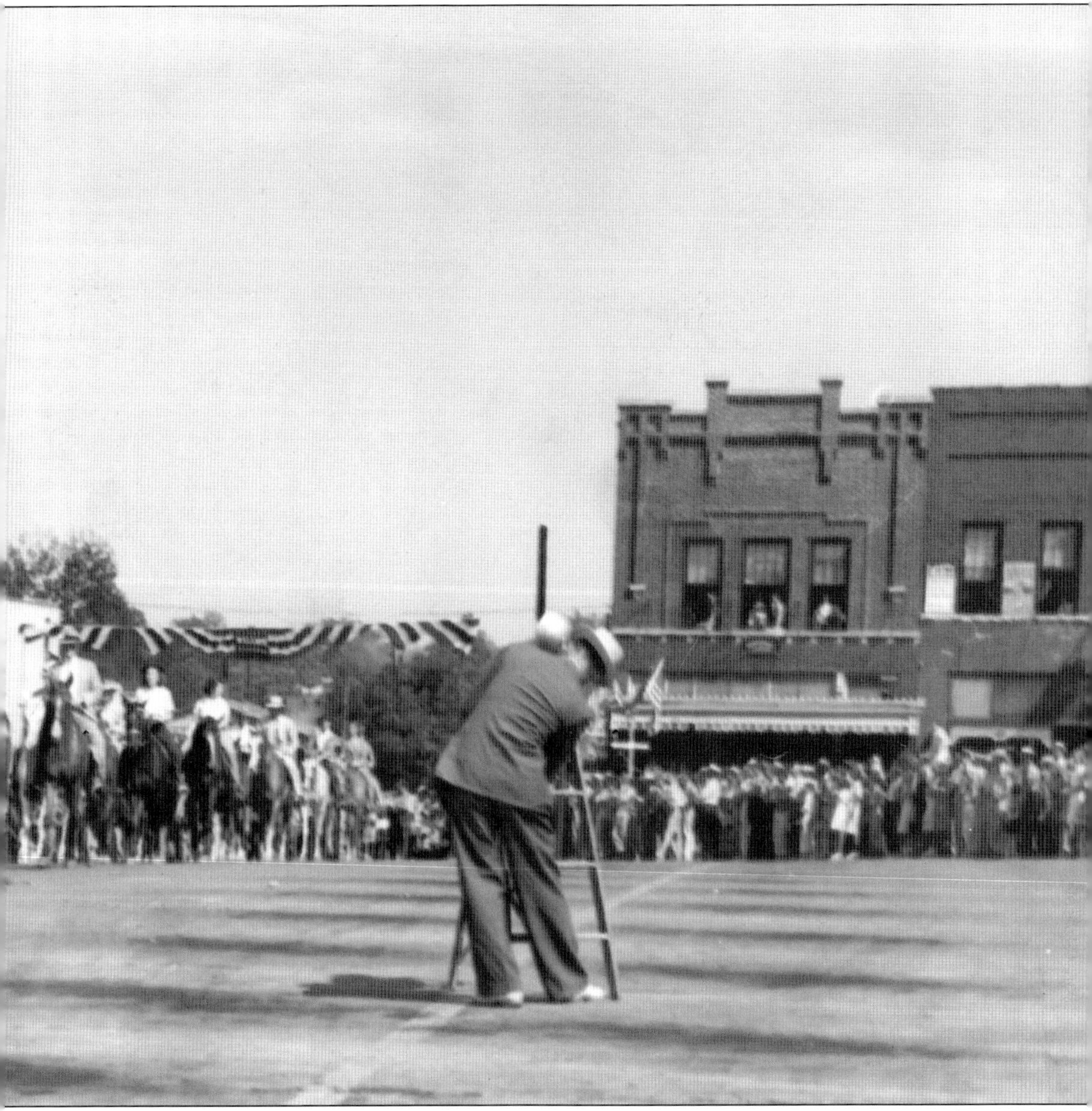

become a major factor in the county's economy. Each year, thousands of trainers, grooms, riders, and owners descend upon the city for the horse show. (Courtesy of Gore Center.)

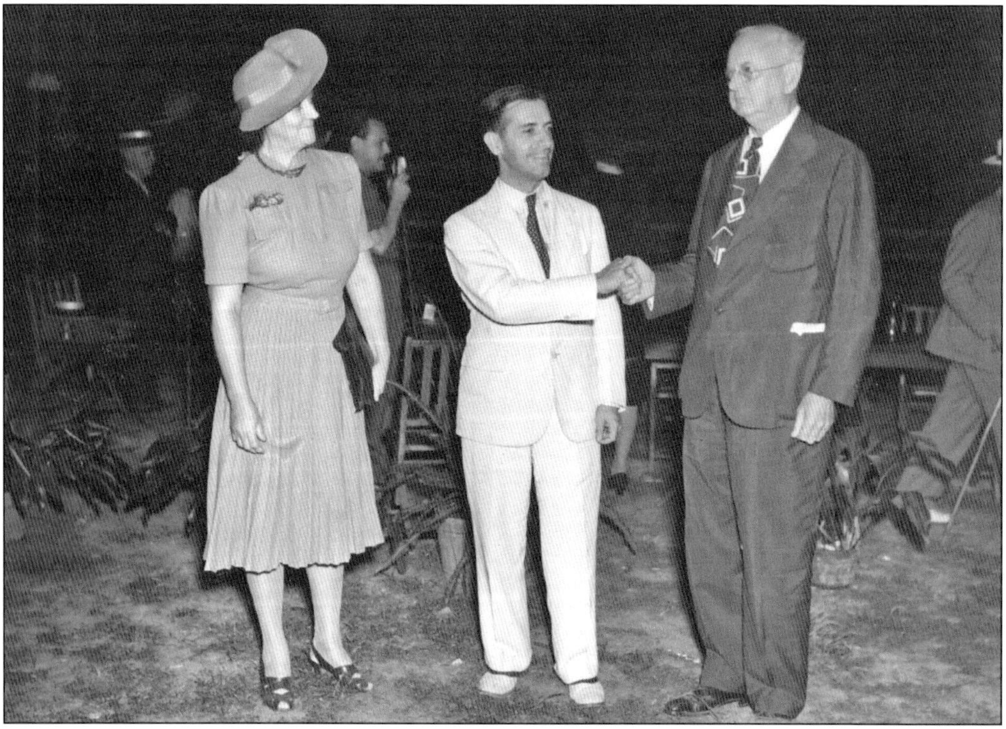

Since its inception, the Celebration has attracted major figures from local and state politics. In this photograph, Col. C. H. Cooper (right) and his wife greet Gov. Prentice Cooper. Each evening's activities provided ample opportunity for spectators and participants to mingle. (Courtesy of Gore Center.)

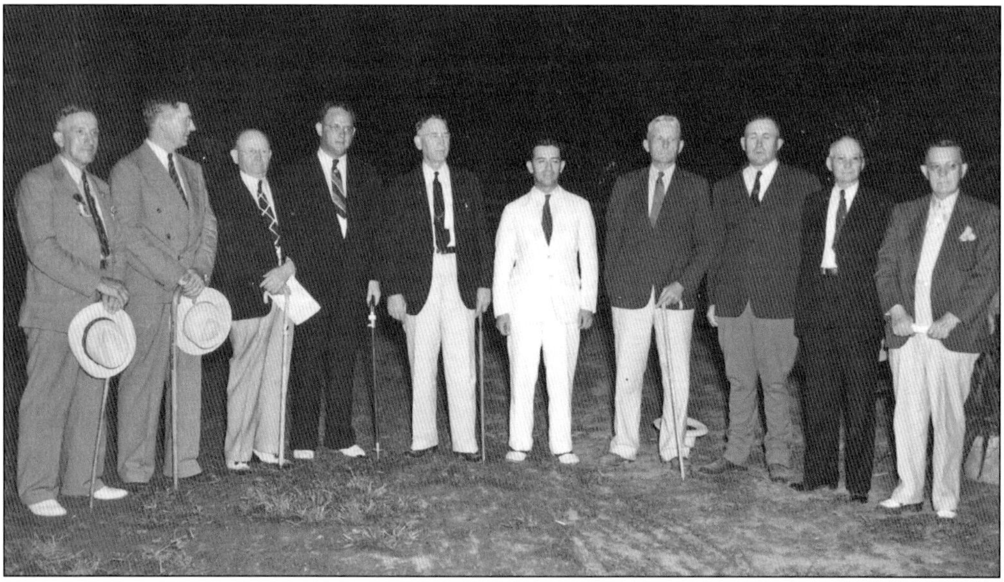

This group of officials at one of the 1939–1945 Tennessee Walking Horse National Celebrations has gathered around Gov. Prentice Cooper (in the center, wearing the white suit). Managing the Celebration, as well as other similar horse shows, required a large staff, including secretaries, announcers, ribbon presenters, gate keepers, and ring stewards. (Courtesy of Gore Center.)

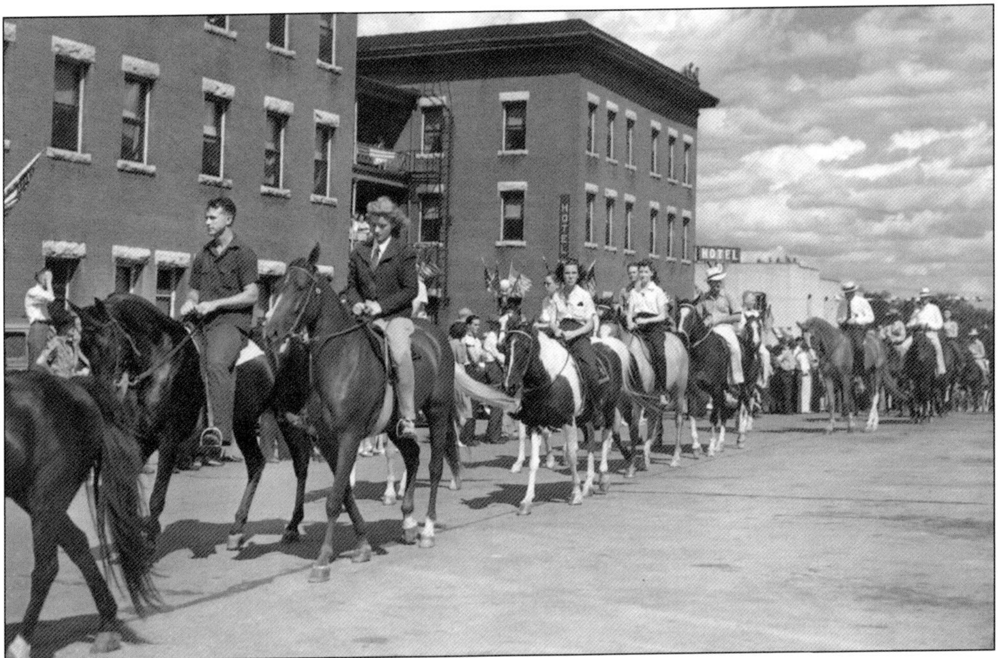

This group of Walking Horses and their riders is presumably part of an early-1940s Tennessee Walking Horse National Celebration parade in Shelbyville. The horses in the middle with the partially white coats are early predecessors of the extremely popular Spotted Saddle Horses, a breed registry that overlaps with the Tennessee Walking Horse registry. (Courtesy of Gore Center.)

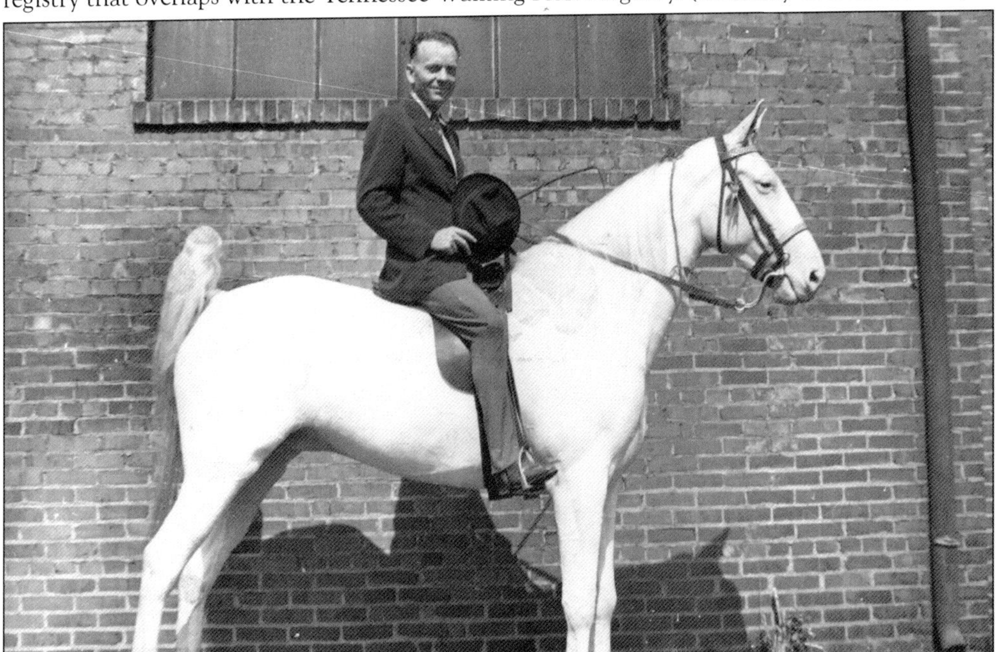

The winner of the 1939 Oldsmobile-Boyds Trophy and runner-up to Strolling Jim was Lillie White, a cremello or "dominant white" mare, ridden in this photograph by D. H. Brock of Lawrenceburg. The mare exemplifies one of the Tennessee Walking Horse's possible color variations. Although not very common, these "white" horses have been quite popular. (Courtesy of Gore Center.)

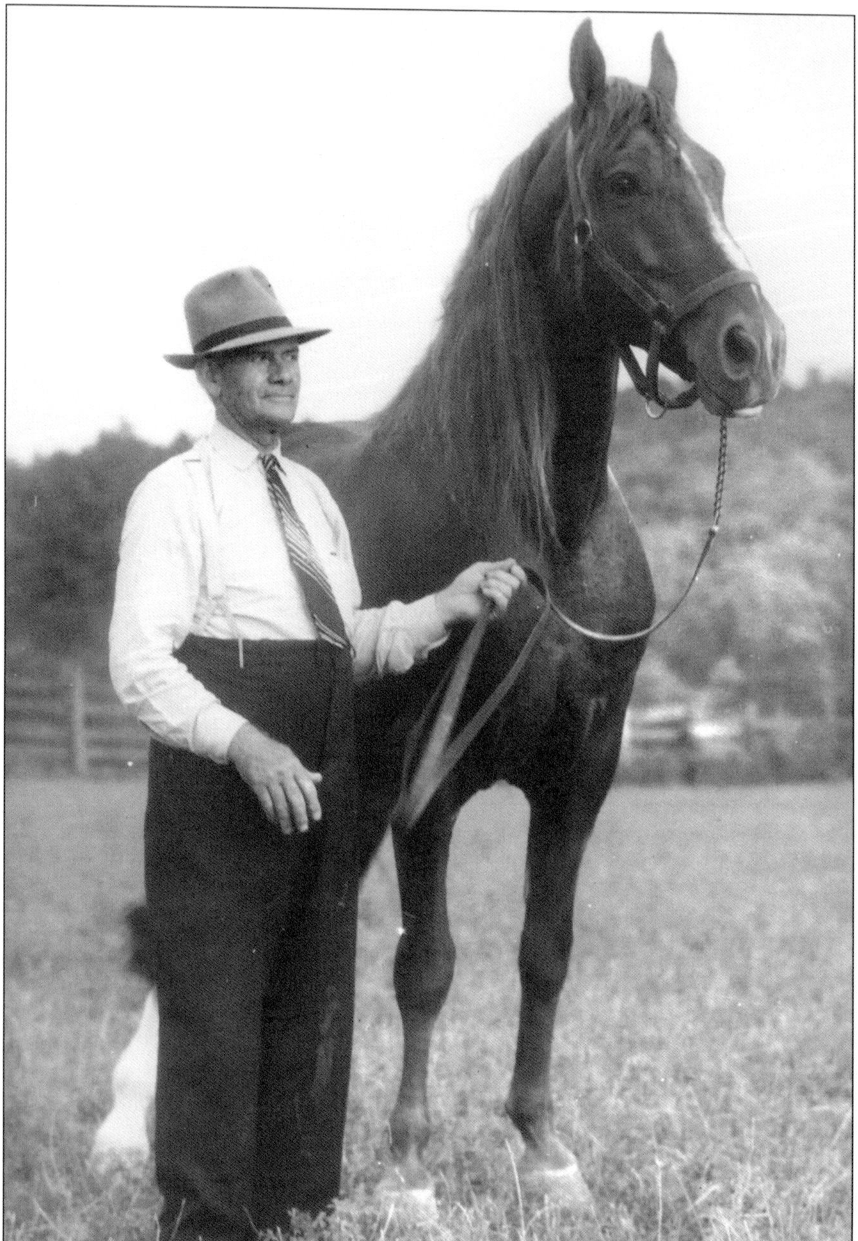

This *c.* 1938 photograph of Hall Allen and his owner, Tom Reynolds Jr., shows a stallion who represents the first foundation horse of the Tennessee Walking Horse breed. Hall Allen's solid build and striking presence are linked to his agricultural and transportation heritage. Hall Allen's most famous sibling was the long-lived (1917–1938) stallion Wilson's Allen 350075. The registration number was important because there were several horses named Wilson's Allen. Wilson's Allen sired over 480 foals, including the first three Grand Champions. Some of Wilson's Allen's offspring include Strolling Jim, Melody Maid, Haynes Peacock, Wilson's Ace, and Midnight Sun. Wilson's Allen was bred by Bud Messick in Coffee County at the urging of Johnson Hill, who purchased the colt. Hill's nephew, a boy named Steve Hill, broke Wilson's Allen to the saddle. He later became a noted trainer. (Courtesy of Gore Center.)

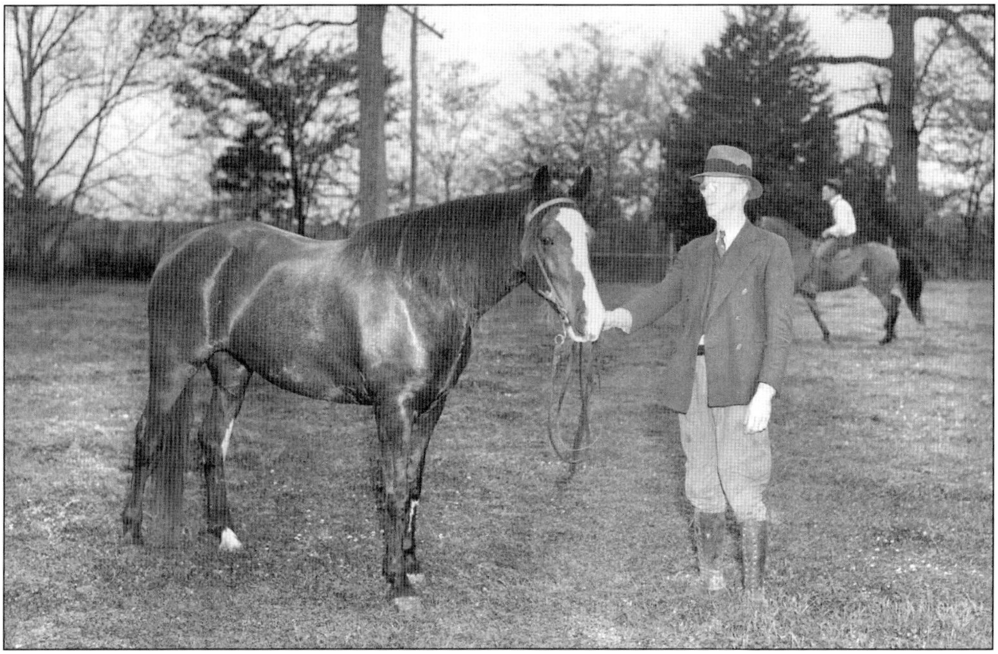

This conformation photograph (used to illustrate a horse's figure) shows the broodmare Beauty, one of many Tennessee Walkers owned by Walter William Ogilvie, an early supporter of the breed. Ogilvie owned Maple Crest Farm, a 515-acre Tennessee century farm (a family farm continuously operated for 100 years) located in College Grove, until his death in 1977. (Courtesy of TSLA.)

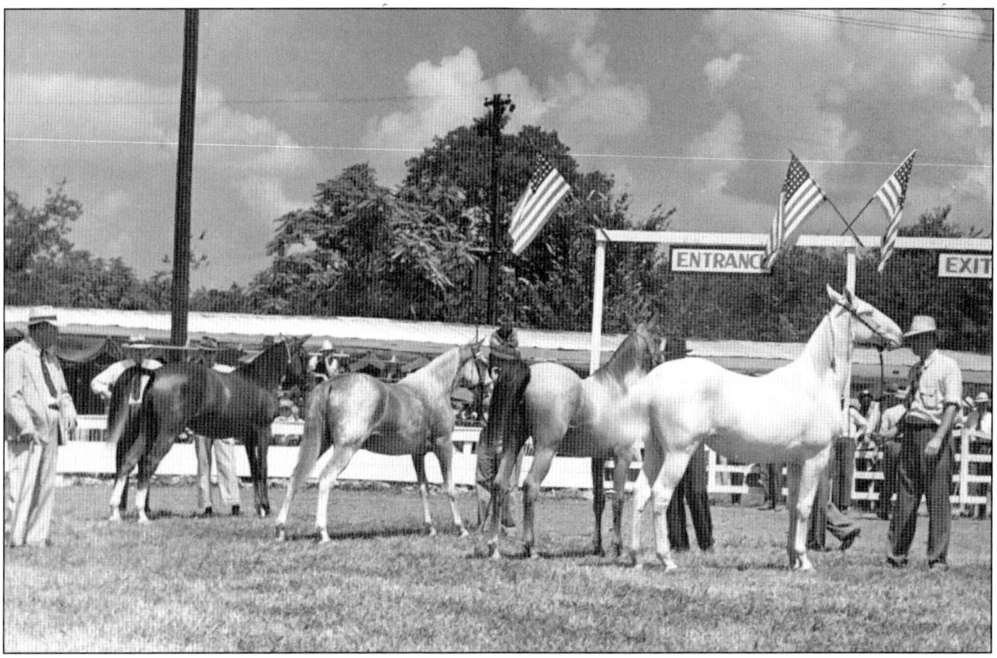

This 1940 photograph shows four two- or three-year-old fillies being judged in the old Tennessee Walking Horse National Celebration show grounds in Shelbyville. Mares are as just important as stallions when breeding horses, and some mares became well known for their successful offspring. (Courtesy of Gore Center.)

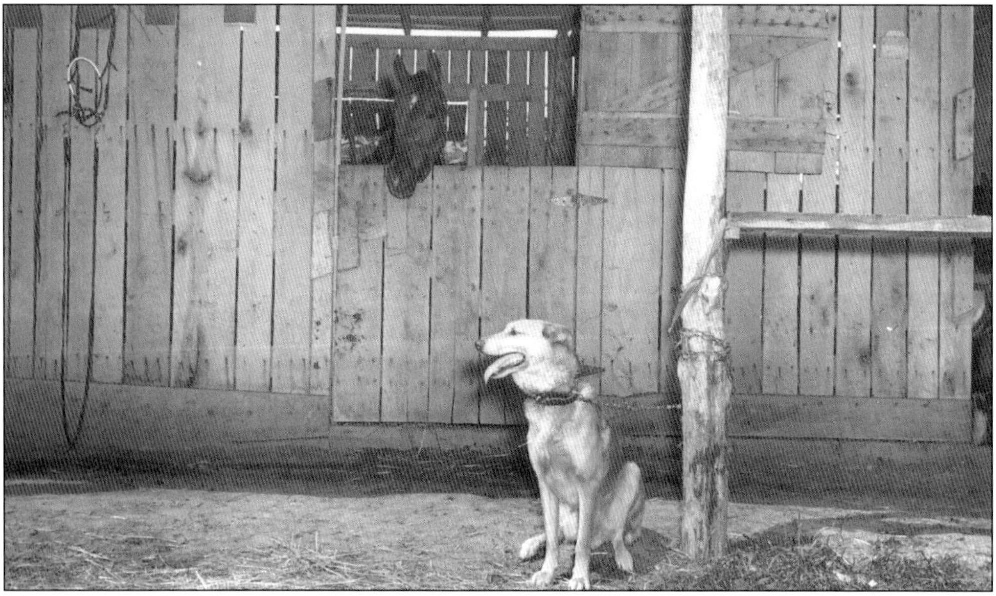

This June 1940 image captures the personality of the first Grand Champion, Strolling Jim, as he looks over his stall door at his watchdog Chum. Taken at Henry Davis's stable in Wartrace, this photograph also hints at the stardom of Tennessee Walking Horses in Middle Tennessee. (Courtesy of TSLA.)

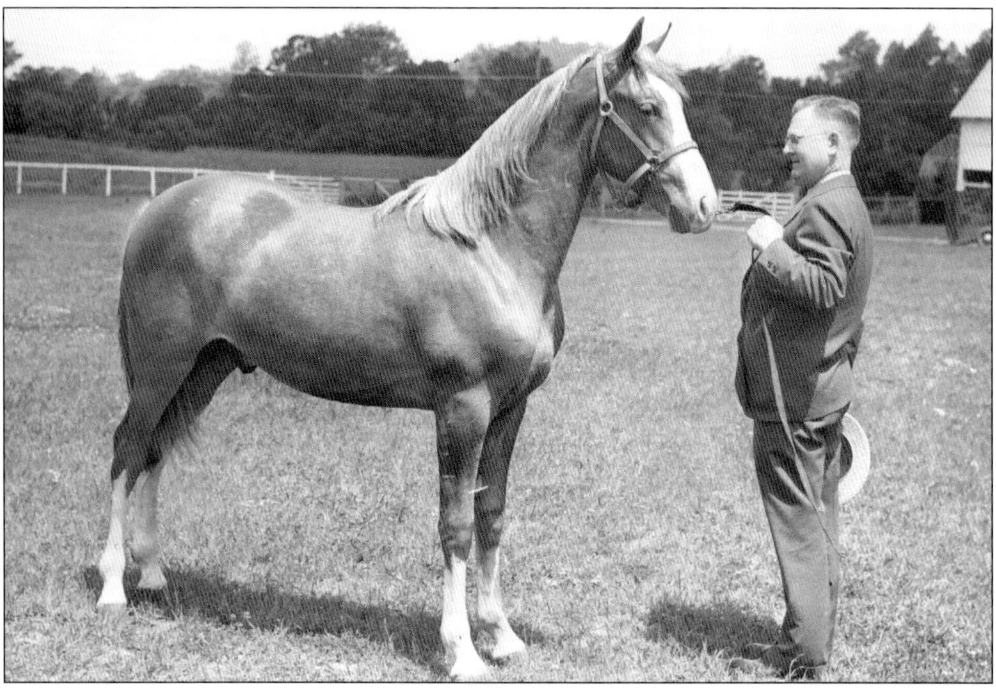

Wirt Harlin, shown in this 1940s photograph with one of his yearlings, established Harlinsdale Farm in Franklin in 1935. He immediately began to build a property that would reflect his success through its "careful landscaping," as described by the Center for Historic Preservation in the property's National Register nomination, and attract potential buyers to the centrally located stable. (Courtesy of TSLA.)

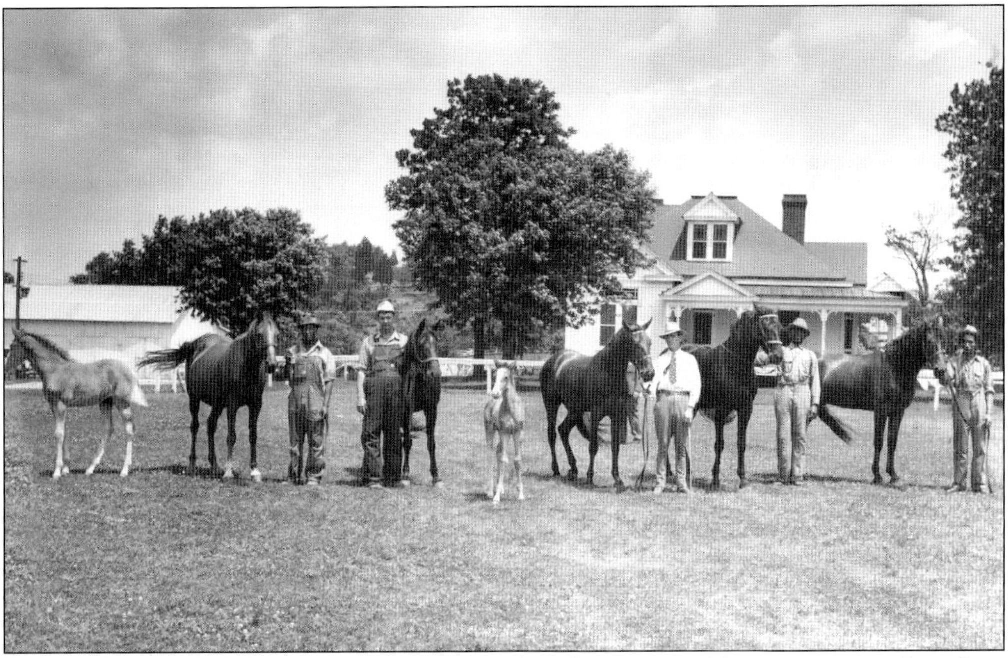

The Harlinsdale livestock had ample pastures with well-constructed fences to protect them from the traffic of Franklin Road, which led into Franklin. Harlinsdale's layout became a template for other 1940s Tennessee Walking Horse breeders and owners who wanted to build new facilities to accommodate the rapidly popularized breed. (Courtesy of TSLA.)

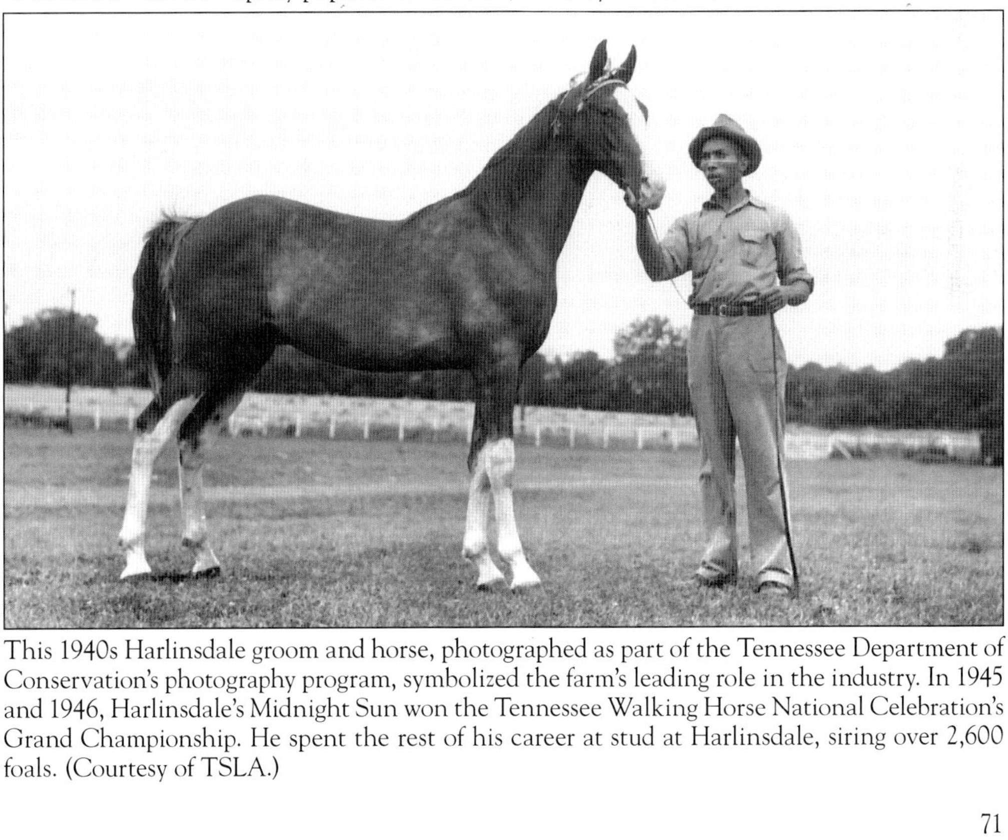

This 1940s Harlinsdale groom and horse, photographed as part of the Tennessee Department of Conservation's photography program, symbolized the farm's leading role in the industry. In 1945 and 1946, Harlinsdale's Midnight Sun won the Tennessee Walking Horse National Celebration's Grand Championship. He spent the rest of his career at stud at Harlinsdale, siring over 2,600 foals. (Courtesy of TSLA.)

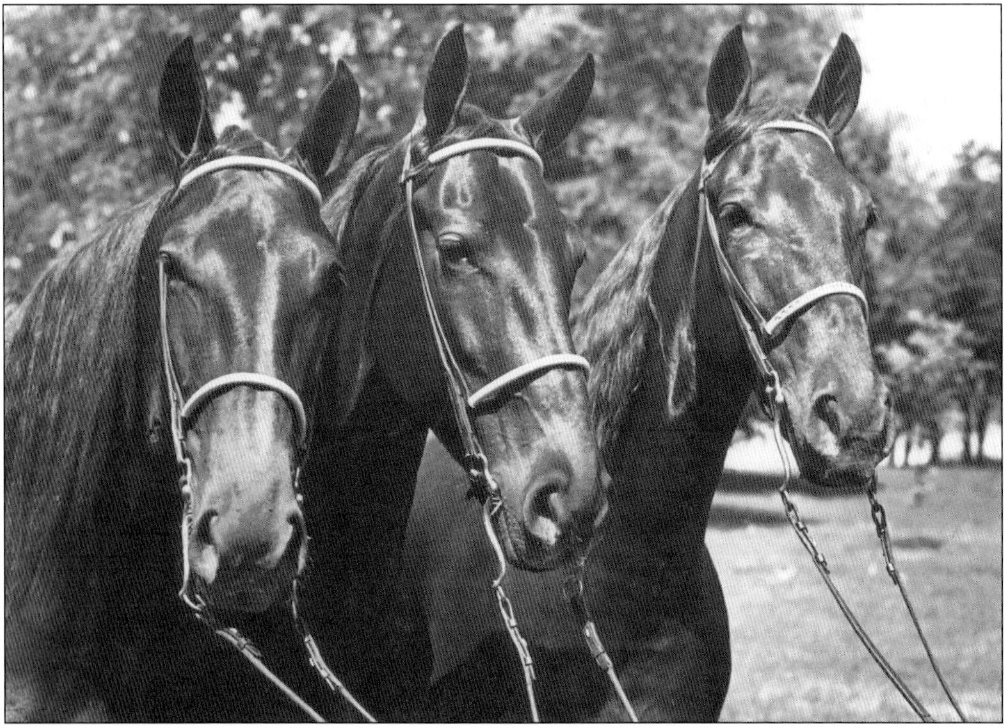

This April 29, 1941, picture shows three prospective champion Tennessee Walking Horses at Oakwood Acres in Fayetteville. The stable's most famous horse was Melody Maid 390812, a chestnut mare who finished her successful career at age five, when Floyd Carothers rode her to the Grand Championship at the 1942 celebration. Melody Maid was the first mare to win Grand Champion. (Courtesy of TSLA.)

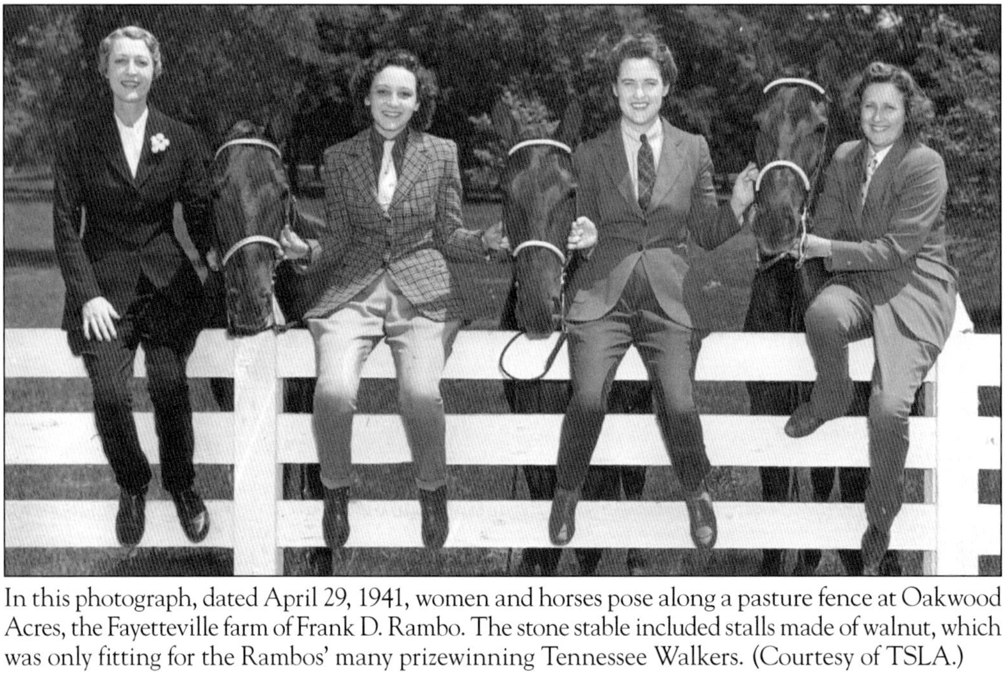

In this photograph, dated April 29, 1941, women and horses pose along a pasture fence at Oakwood Acres, the Fayetteville farm of Frank D. Rambo. The stone stable included stalls made of walnut, which was only fitting for the Rambos' many prizewinning Tennessee Walkers. (Courtesy of TSLA.)

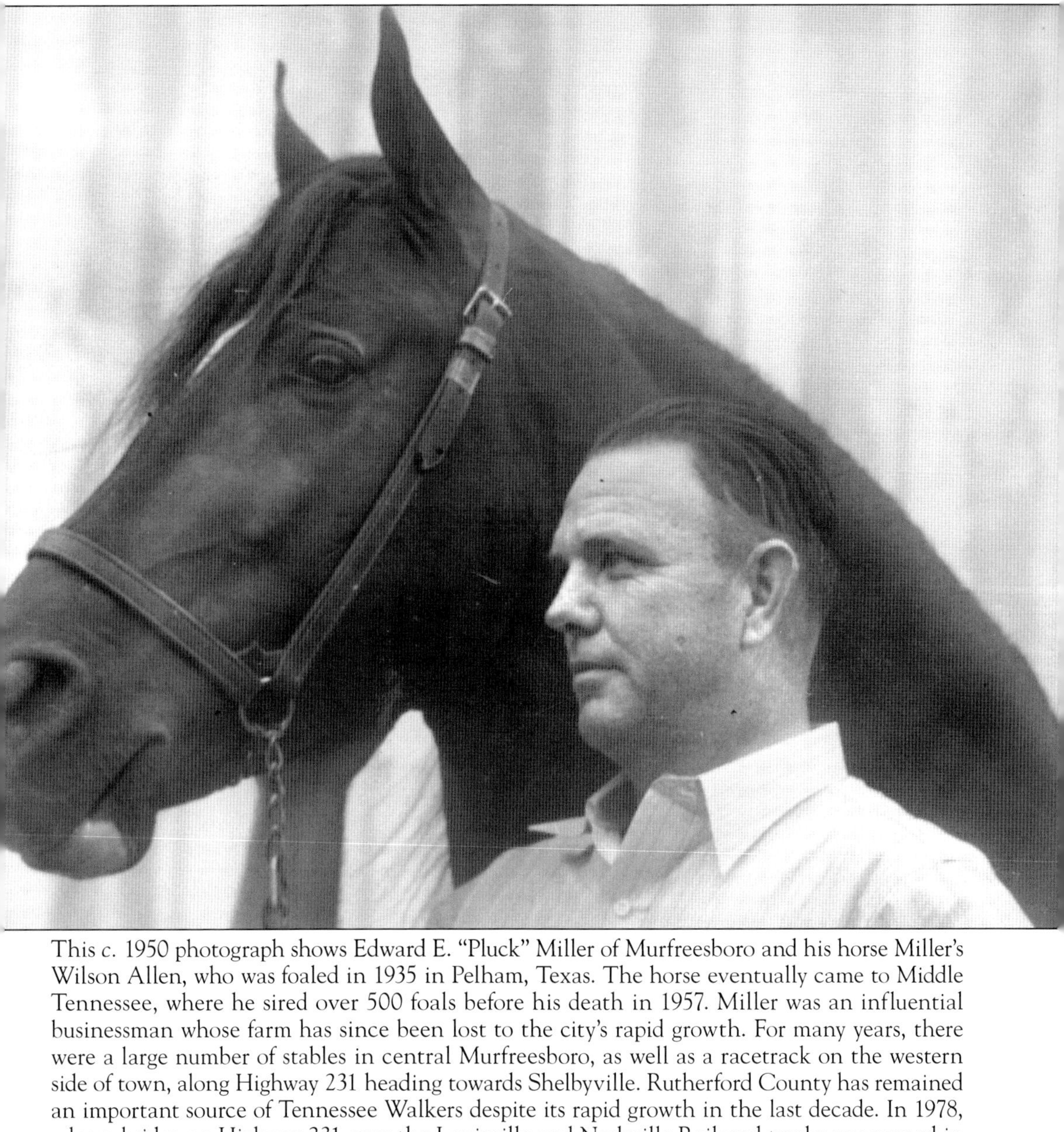

This *c.* 1950 photograph shows Edward E. "Pluck" Miller of Murfreesboro and his horse Miller's Wilson Allen, who was foaled in 1935 in Pelham, Texas. The horse eventually came to Middle Tennessee, where he sired over 500 foals before his death in 1957. Miller was an influential businessman whose farm has since been lost to the city's rapid growth. For many years, there were a large number of stables in central Murfreesboro, as well as a racetrack on the western side of town, along Highway 231 heading towards Shelbyville. Rutherford County has remained an important source of Tennessee Walkers despite its rapid growth in the last decade. In 1978, a large bridge on Highway 231 over the Louisville and Nashville Railroad tracks was named in Miller's honor. (Courtesy of Gore Center.)

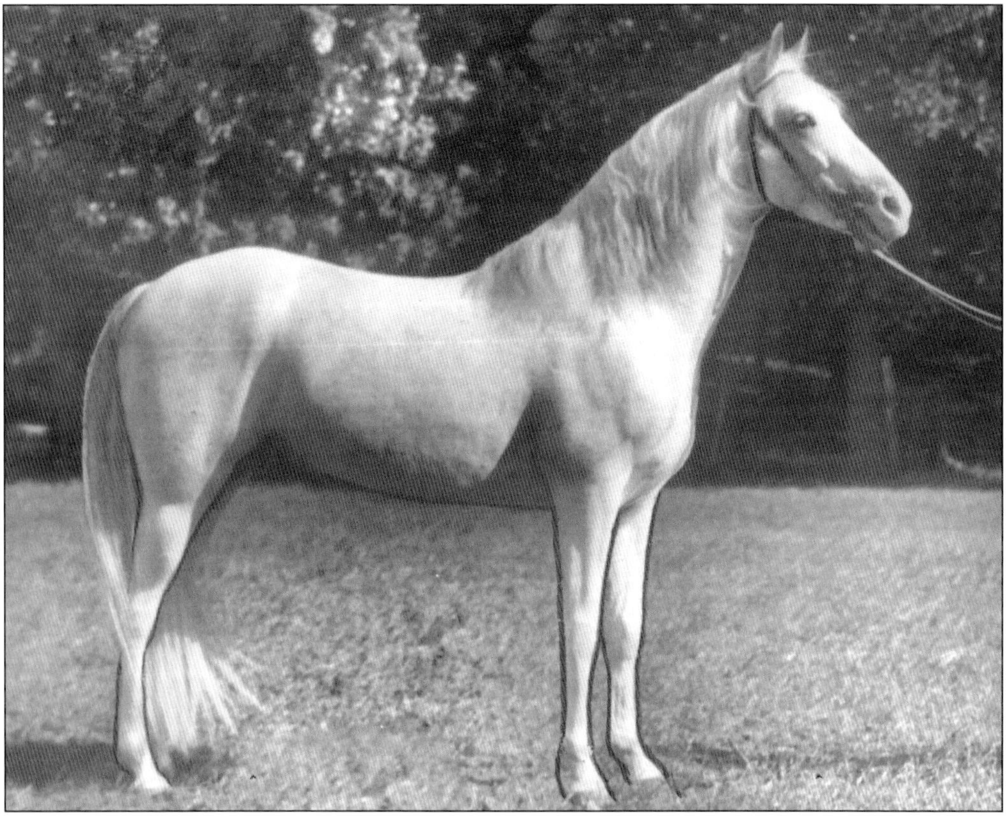

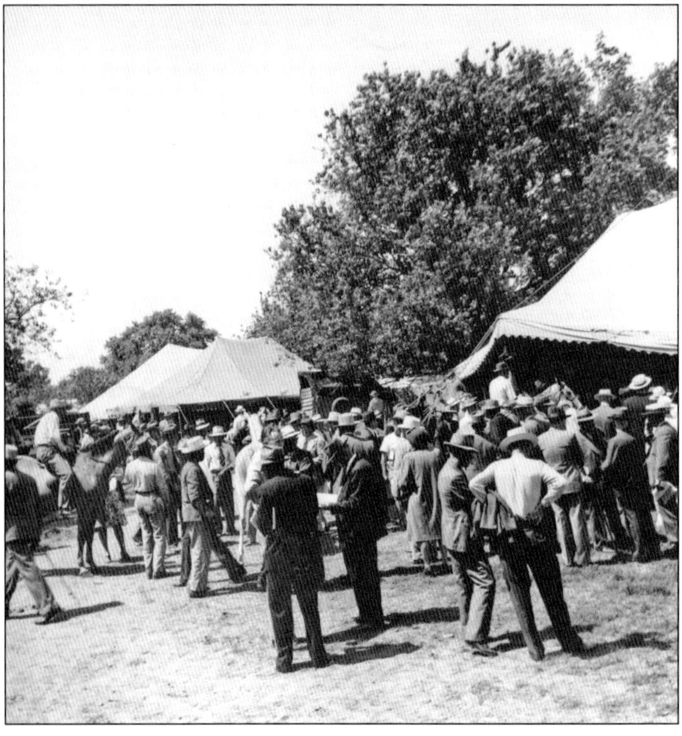

John W. Taylor of Eagleville owned the horse featured in this conformation photograph, Captain Eddie, who was sired by Merry Boy out of (mothered by) Grace Darling. This horse was one of the many grandsons of the foundation sire Roan Allen F-38, to whom almost all Tennessee Walking Horses today can be traced. (Courtesy of Gore Center.)

This 1950s photograph of a Murray Farm Walking Horse sale shows the popularity of annual farm sales and the excitement surrounding them. The auction took place under the tents. A single horse truck is parked between the tents. (Courtesy of Gore Center.)

Five

1906–1945

The four decades from 1906 to 1945 saw a significant change in the breeding and use of horses in Middle Tennessee. No longer were breeders focused on producing large numbers of horses meant for a single purpose, as had farms like Belle Meade, Hermitage Stud, and Fairview in the previous century. Instead, they began to produce horses with the ability to participate in a wider range of activities. As Middle Tennesseans prospered during the 1910s and 1920s, they created a society that reaffirmed the value of equestrian skills and knowledge. Thanks to rapidly expanding recreational choices and newly available older breeds, such as the Arabian, horsemen (and women) began to plan year-long schedules filled with horse shows, races, and foxhunts.

In the early years of the 20th century, horse shows began to slowly change, becoming competitive events that represented the pinnacle of each breed and sport. In the past, horse shows had usually been part of larger fairs, with classes for all types of horses. The new horse shows provided a venue for breeders and trainers to compare horses, exchange training methods, and develop standards for the breeds and sports. Spectators needed to be fully versed in the particular type of horse that they were watching in order to fully appreciate the competition.

Steeplechasing continued the specialization trend but built upon the area's older flat racing tradition. By the late 1920s, there were several steeplechase courses, used for racing Thoroughbreds over fences, in Middle Tennessee. In 1936, the Works Progress Administration built a steeplechase course and buildings for a riding academy at Nashville's Edwin Warner Park. The first Iroquois Steeplechase, named for the famed Belle Meade stallion, was run in 1941.

Other sporting enthusiasts, often the same ones who participated in steeplechasing, resumed foxhunting in the areas to the south and west of Nashville. Although several private families, including the Jacksons at Belle Meade, had maintained private foxhound packs in the 19th century, foxhunting did not gain broad popularity until the late 1930s. Filled with British traditions, foxhunting served to reinforce social status through the display of equestrian skills and etiquette.

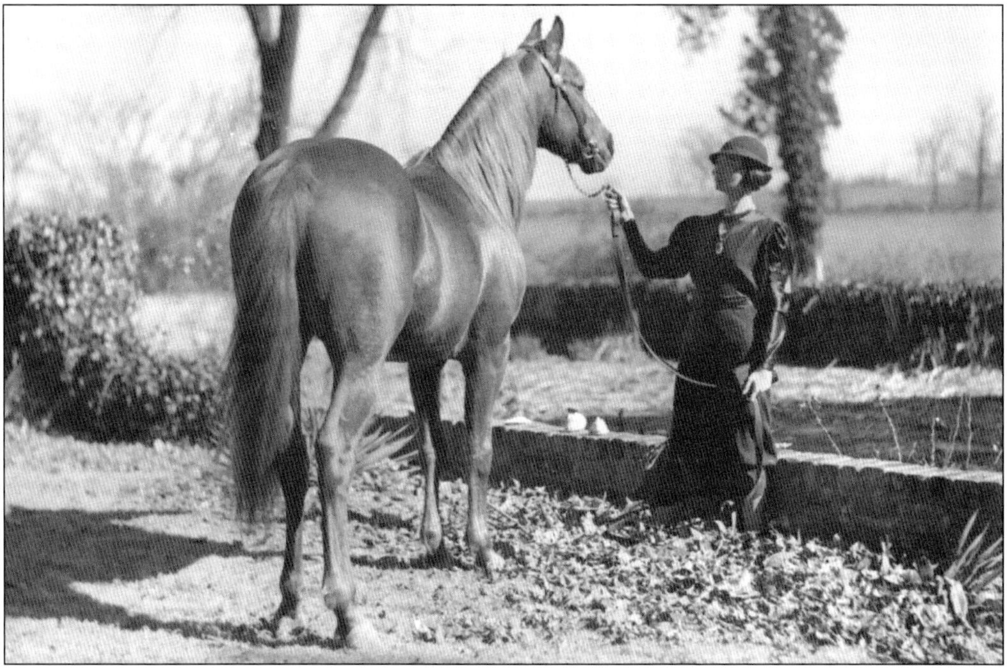

Above, Margaret Lindsley Warden and Travellers Rest's Arabian stallion Antez stand in front of the estate's garden in the 1920s. Warden contributed more to the recreational and sporting popularity of horses in Middle Tennessee than did any other individual in the 20th century. A native Nashvillian, Warden began writing editorial columns about equestrian activities for the *Tennessean* under the pseudonym Cade (the name of a famous English Thoroughbred) in 1925. In 1939, she began a 55-year-long career writing a Sunday column, "Horse Sense," which she used to encourage, educate, inform, and, occasionally, chastise Middle Tennesseans about their horse-related activities. Below is an image of the Arabian stallion Bazleyd, owned by Warden's cousin Jacob McGavock Dickinson Jr., at his stud Travellers Rest. (Courtesy of Gore Center.)

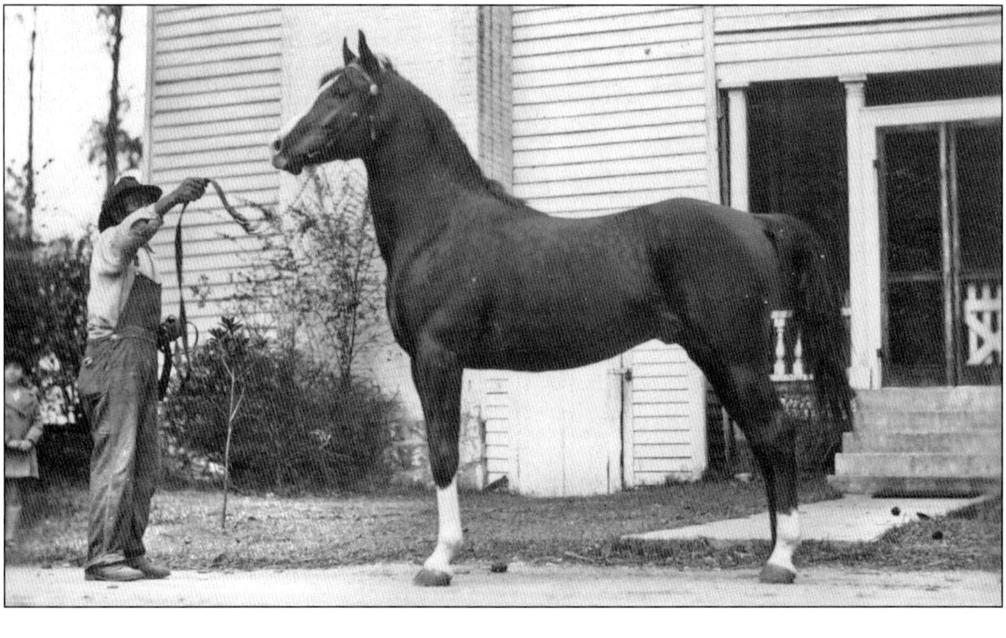

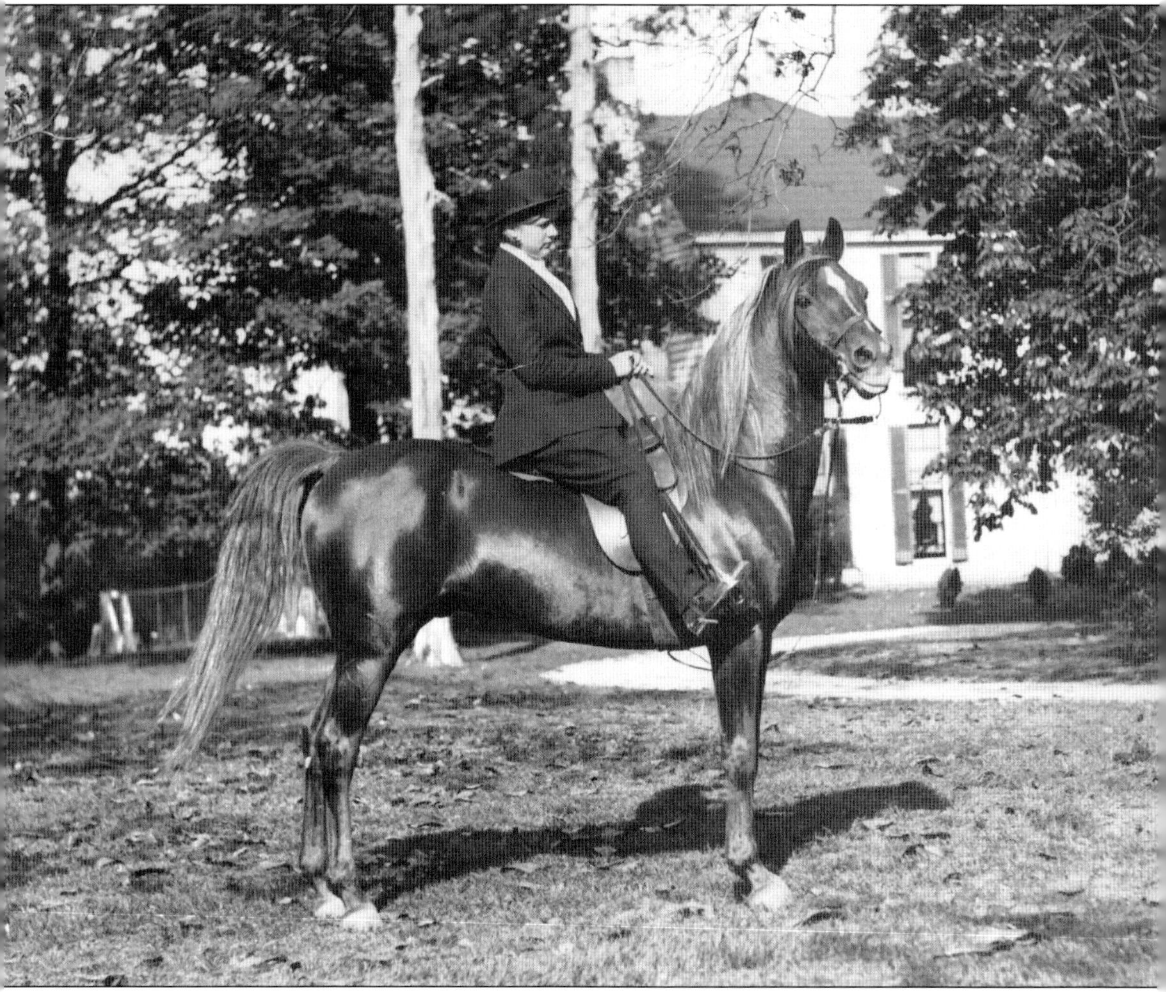

This c. 1930 photograph of Peggy Dickinson and her family's Arabian stallion Antez was taken in Nashville next to their historic home, Travellers Rest, which was established by John Overton in 1799. Antez was one of the Dickinsons' most successful horses: He raced at Cumberland Park, and he was the champion of the Tennessee State Fair's horse shows in 1927 and 1928. In 1934, Dickinson sold Antez to the Polish stud to help reestablish Arabian breeding in Poland, which had been disrupted by the wars of the late 19th and early 20th centuries. Travellers Rest's Arabians were prized for their pure bloodlines, and the farm quickly grew to be the largest Arabian stud in the entire South. In 1953, Peggy Dickinson reestablished Travellers Rest Stud on a historic farm outside of Columbia, where she continued her father's tradition of breeding high-quality, versatile horses. (Courtesy of Travellers Rest Plantation and Museum.)

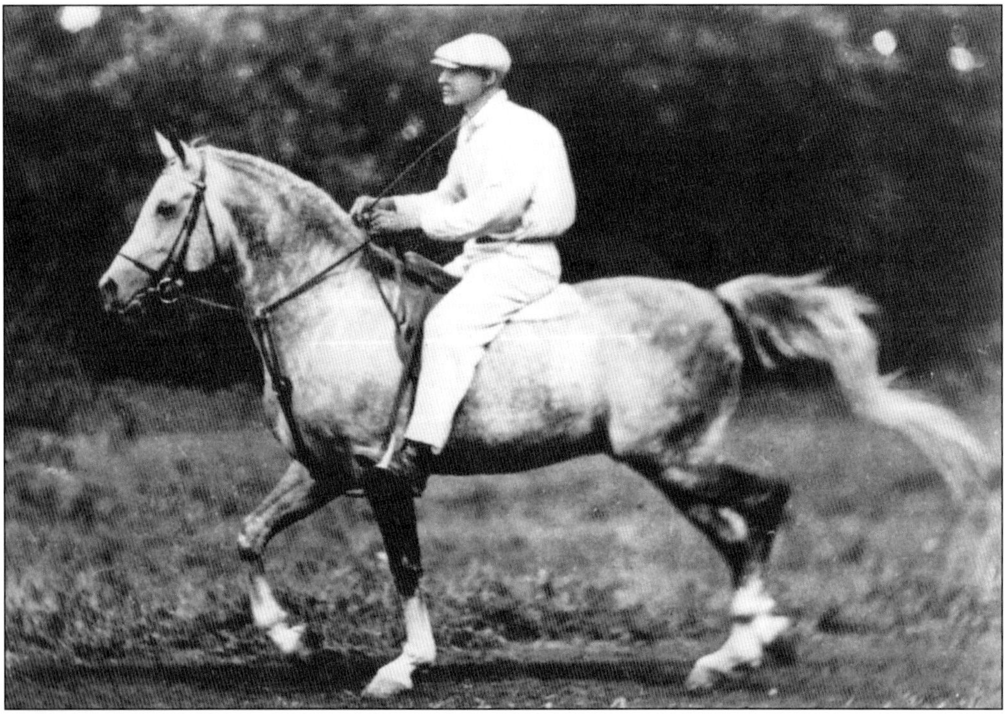

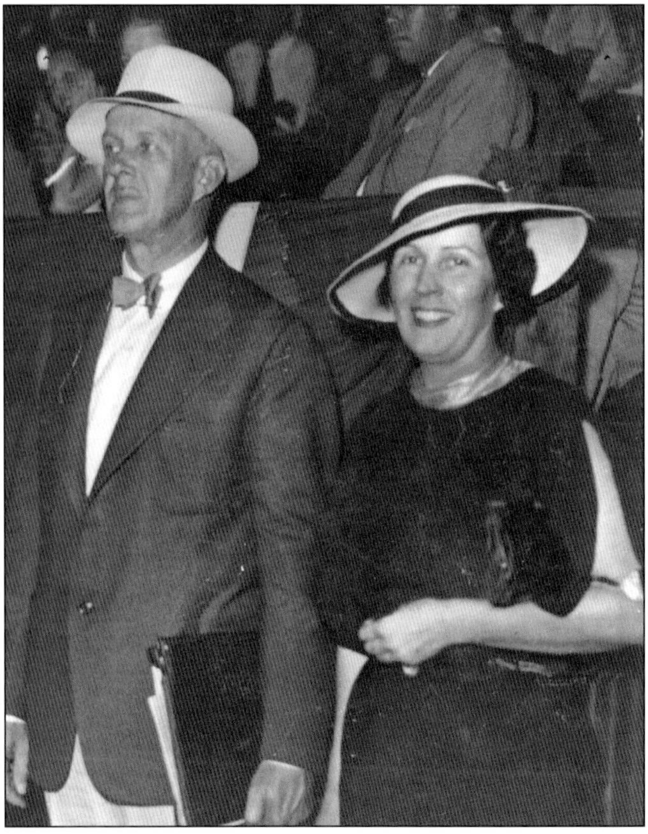

*Zarife, a stallion imported from Egypt in 1932 who then made his way to Travellers Rest, was part of Jacob McGavock Dickinson Jr.'s successful attempt to reestablish the Arabian in the United States. As part of that effort, Dickinson encouraged the U.S. Remount (a part of the war department) to include Arabians in its breeding program. (Courtesy of Travellers Rest Plantation and Museum.)

In 1930, the renowned artist George Ford Morris was photographed attending the Tennessee State Fair with Margaret Clary. Jacob McGavock Dickinson Jr. of Travellers Rest was instrumental in restarting the fair's horse show. Dickinson commissioned Morris to create portraits of his best Arabians. (Courtesy of Gore Center.)

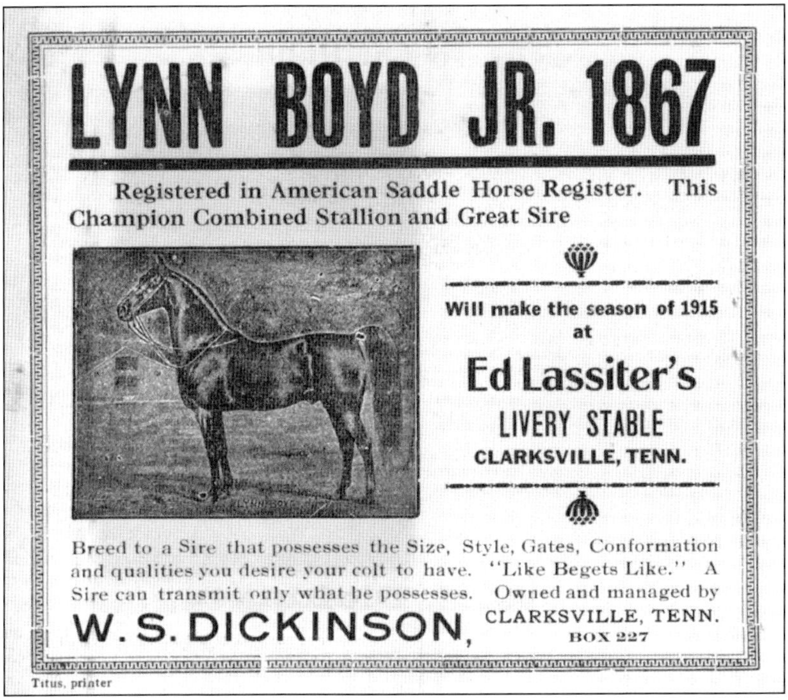
LYNN BOYD JR. 1867
Registered in American Saddle Horse Register. This Champion Combined Stallion and Great Sire
Will make the season of 1915 at
Ed Lassiter's
LIVERY STABLE
CLARKSVILLE, TENN.
Breed to a Sire that possesses the Size, Style, Gates, Conformation and qualities you desire your colt to have. "Like Begets Like." A Sire can transmit only what he possesses. Owned and managed by
W. S. DICKINSON, CLARKSVILLE, TENN. BOX 227
Titus, printer

This 1915 sale bill advertises the black Saddlebred stallion Lynn Boyd Jr. 1867, foaled in 1899. As horse shows proliferated, Middle Tennessee breeders began to buy Kentucky- and Missouri-bred saddle horses to breed for the growing local market. (Courtesy of Gore Center.)

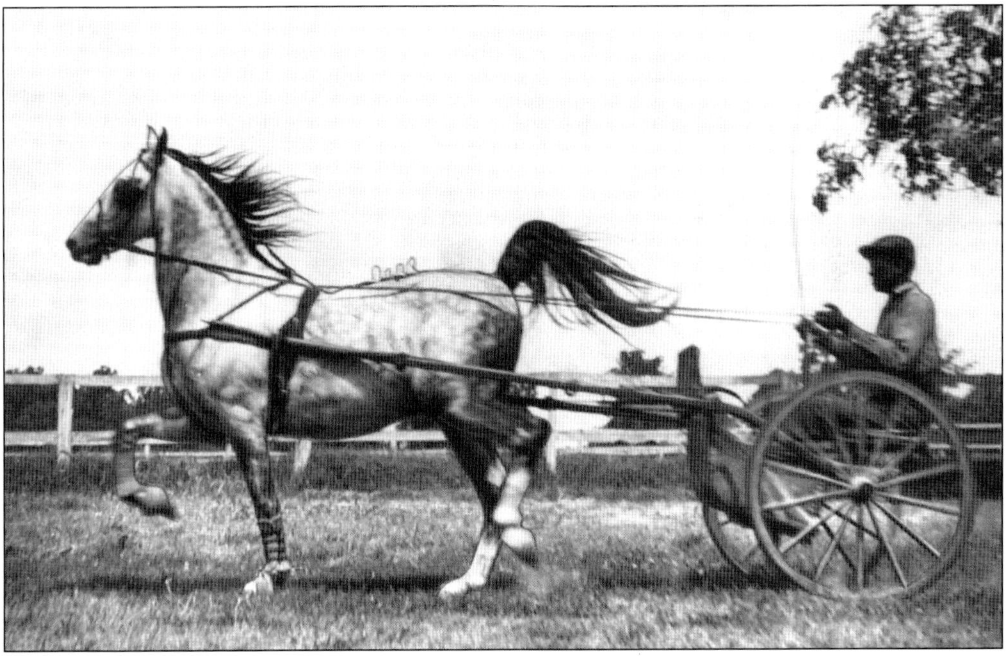

The gray 1934 Saddlebred stallion Tops McDonald, trotting in harness at the West Meade Stable, is shown here in the late 1930s or early 1940s. The McDonald strain is an important foundation line of the Saddlebred. The driver was almost certainly preparing the horse for an area horse show. (Courtesy of Gore Center.)

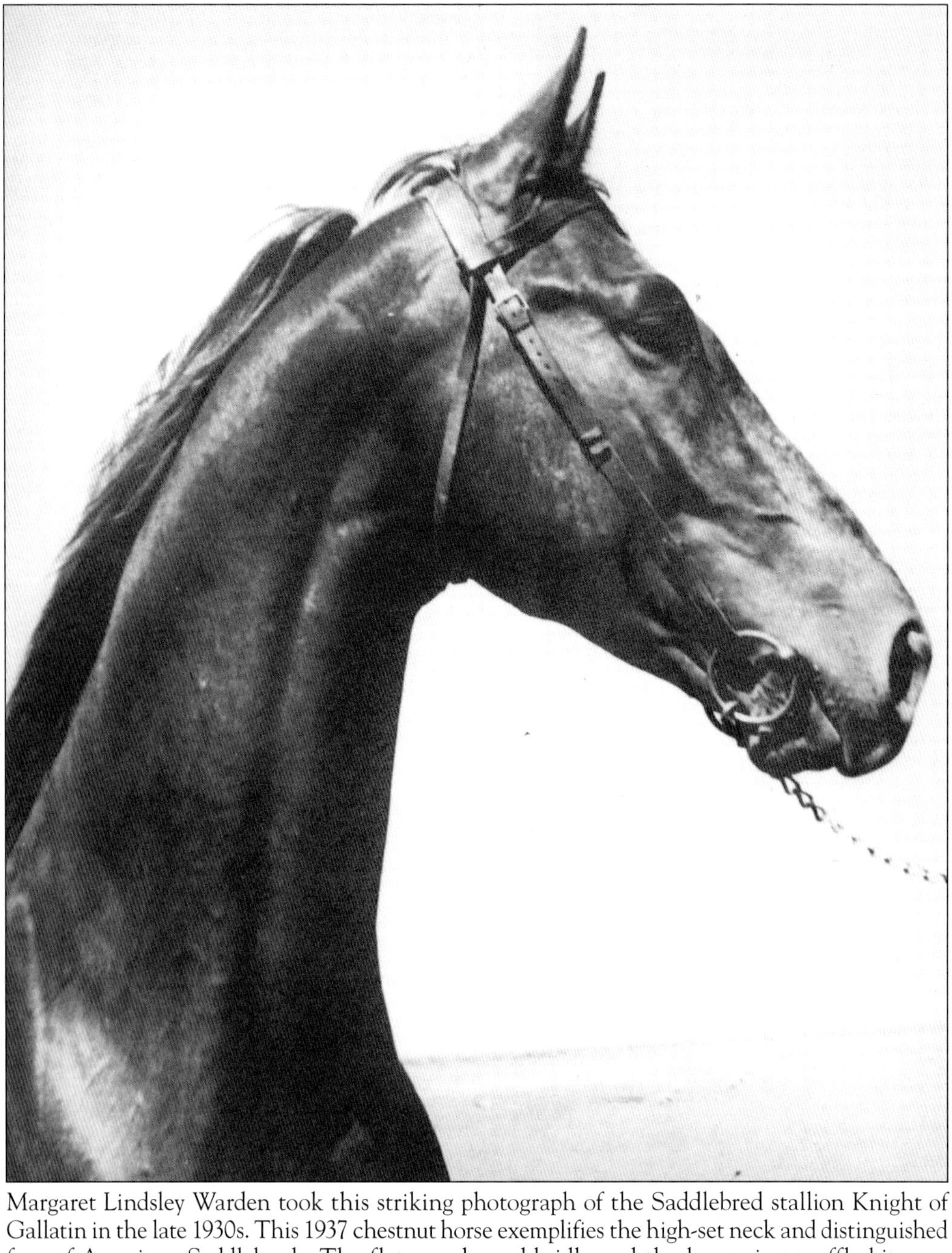

Margaret Lindsley Warden took this striking photograph of the Saddlebred stallion Knight of Gallatin in the late 1930s. This 1937 chestnut horse exemplifies the high-set neck and distinguished face of American Saddlebreds. The flat, unadorned bridle and the loose ring snaffle bit were common of the time period. On his sire's side, Knight of Gallatin traces back to the noted Peavine and Denmark lines and on his dam's side to the Bourbon lines. Saddlebred owners usually exhibited their horses locally until they were ready to travel to Kentucky or Missouri for the nationally recognized Saddlebred competitions. From 1900 to the 1940s, a majority of the Middle Tennessee Saddlebred stables were located north of Nashville. The cities of Lebanon and Gallatin were home to such horses as Red Harrison, Fair Ace King (a U.S. Remount stallion), and Victor Peavine. (Courtesy of Gore Center.)

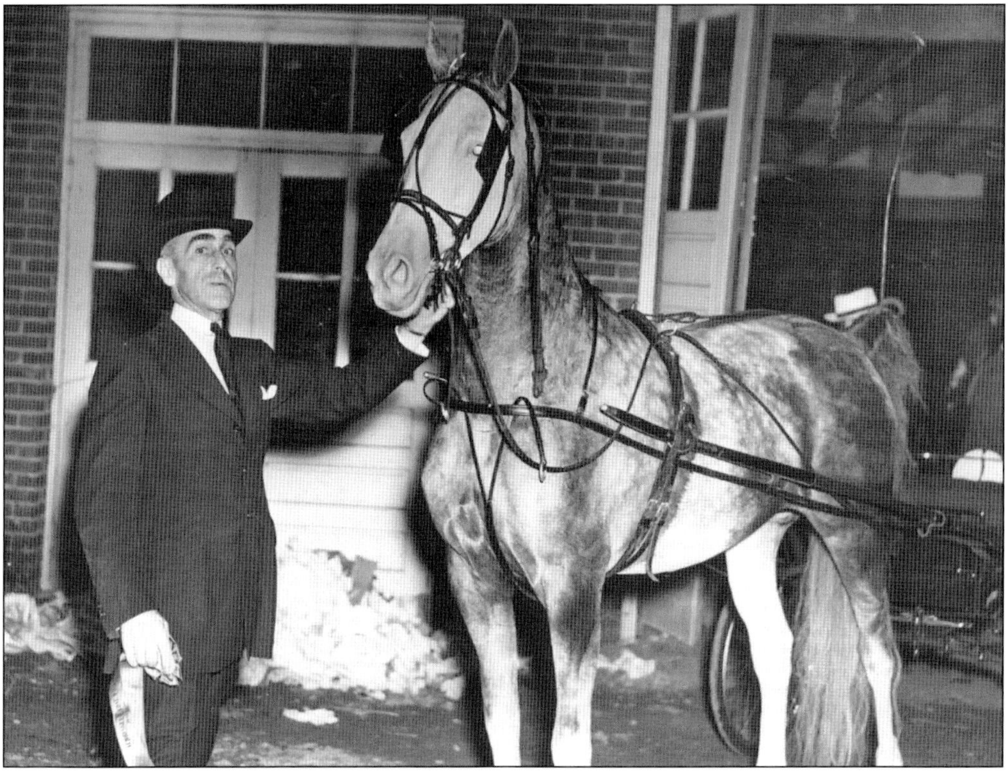

This 1941 photograph shows H. C. Barham with the Saddlebred Heavenly Jane hitched to a cart for either a fine harness or park class, possibly at the state fair. Saddlebreds are often trained to go under saddle (be ridden) and to be driven. (Courtesy of Gore Center.)

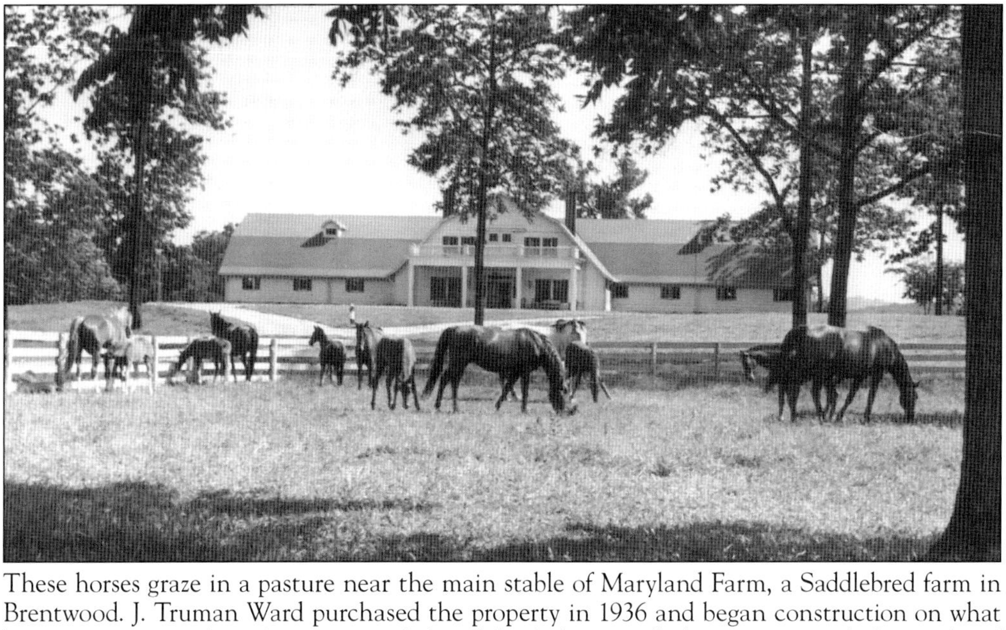

These horses graze in a pasture near the main stable of Maryland Farm, a Saddlebred farm in Brentwood. J. Truman Ward purchased the property in 1936 and began construction on what became a 317-acre showplace surrounded and divided internally by approximately four miles of fencing. (Courtesy of TSLA.)

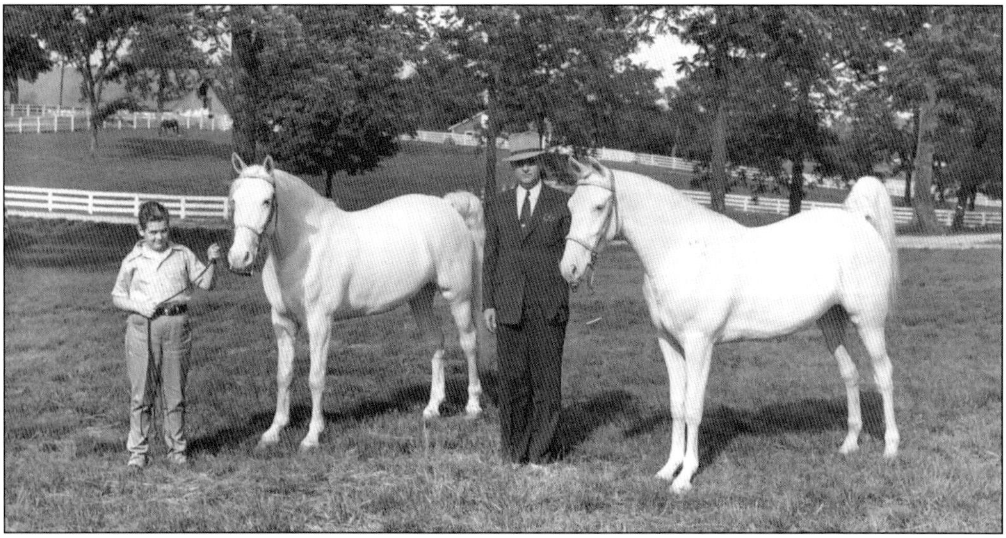

J. Truman Ward and his son, Jimmy, stand with two Saddlebred mares in this *c.* 1941 photograph. In 1941, Ward purchased the nationally known stallion American Ace, along with eight mares, from Spindletop Farm in Lexington, Kentucky. The purchase, as described by Margaret Lindsley Warden in her January 12, 1941, "Horse Sense" column, was "a leap forward for Middle Tennessee's growing fine saddle horse industry." (Courtesy of TSLA.)

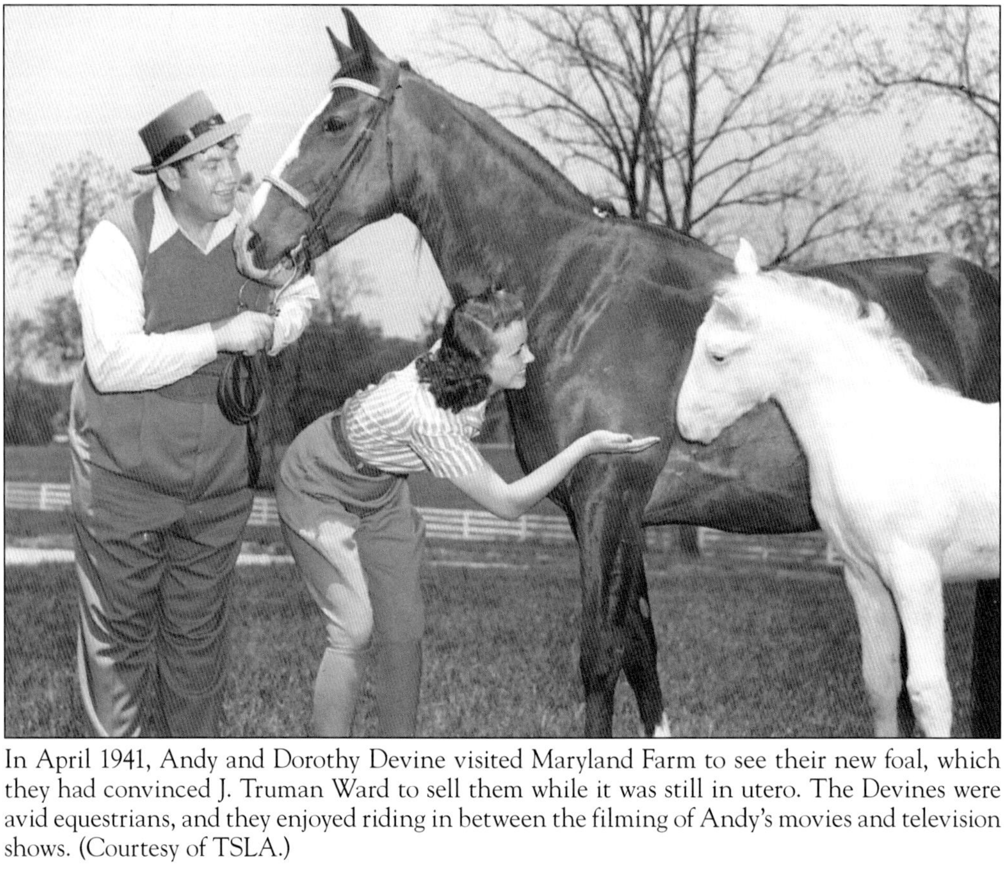

In April 1941, Andy and Dorothy Devine visited Maryland Farm to see their new foal, which they had convinced J. Truman Ward to sell them while it was still in utero. The Devines were avid equestrians, and they enjoyed riding in between the filming of Andy's movies and television shows. (Courtesy of TSLA.)

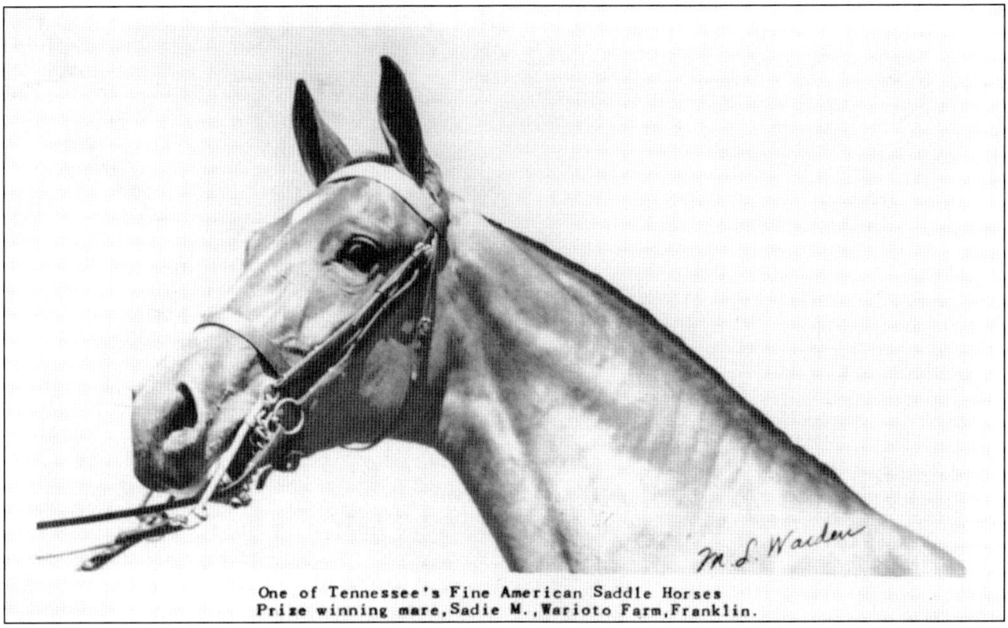

Sadie M., a bay 1939 Saddlebred mare, is seen in this 1948 photograph. She won the 1939 Tennessee State Fair's Breeders' Futurity Championship. Her trainer was Ed Stalcup, and her owner was Joe Werthan of Warioto Farm in Franklin. (Courtesy of Gore Center.)

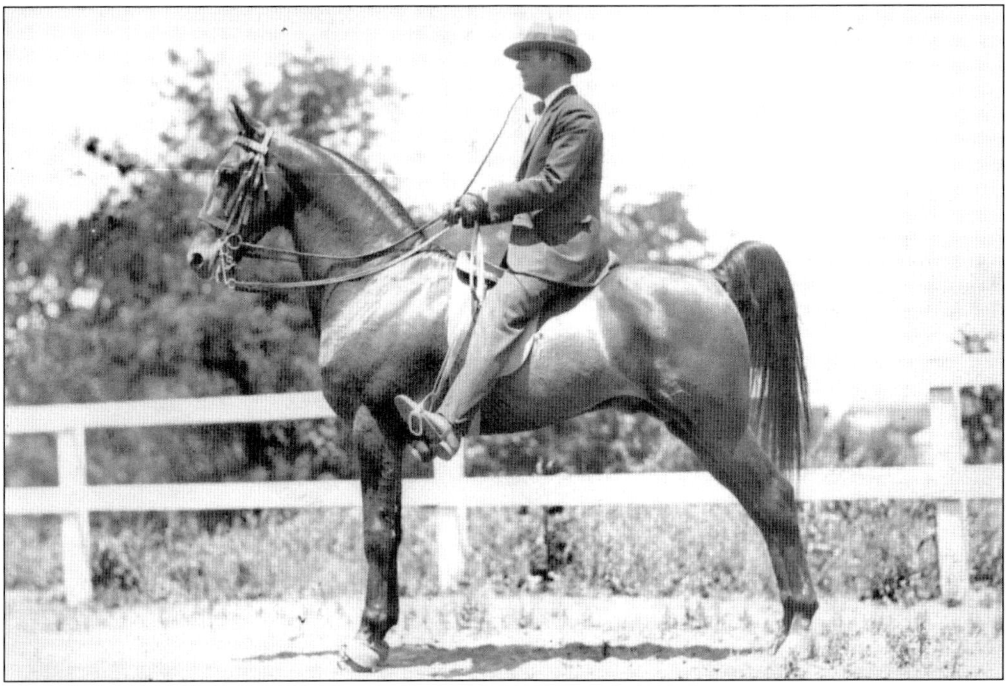
Ed Stalcup, a well-known Middle Tennessee trainer of the early 20th century, is shown here on Golden Rod, owned by Dr. W. D. Haggard of Nashville. This photograph was most likely taken at an outdoor horse show. These shows were extremely popular in the spring and summer months. (Courtesy of Gore Center.)

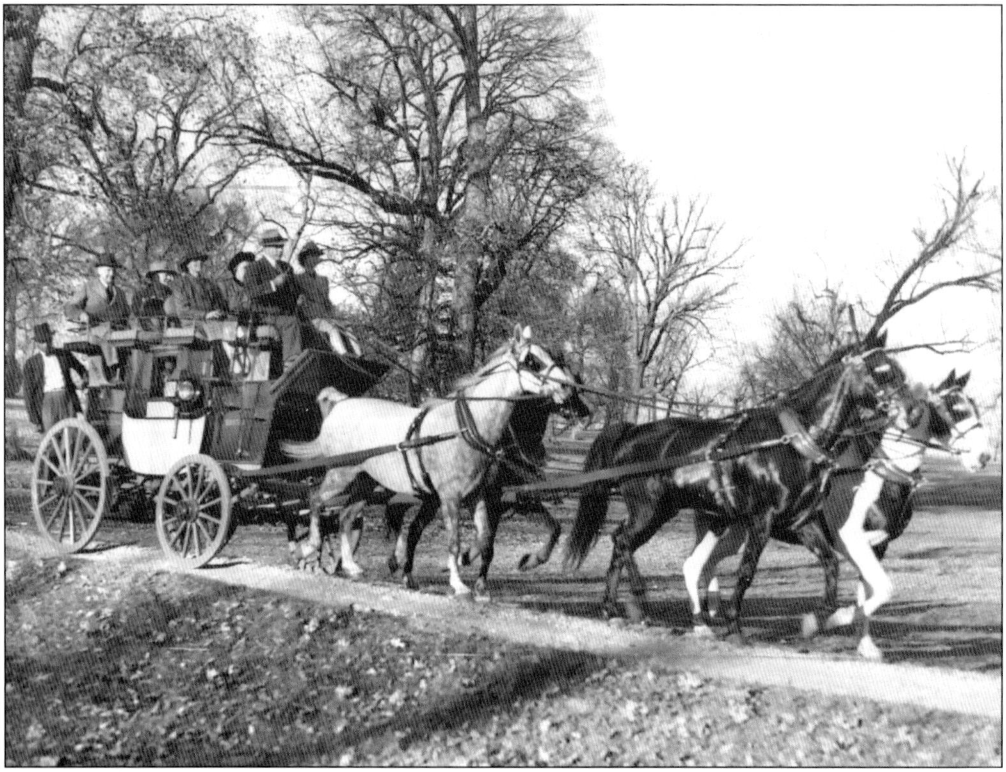

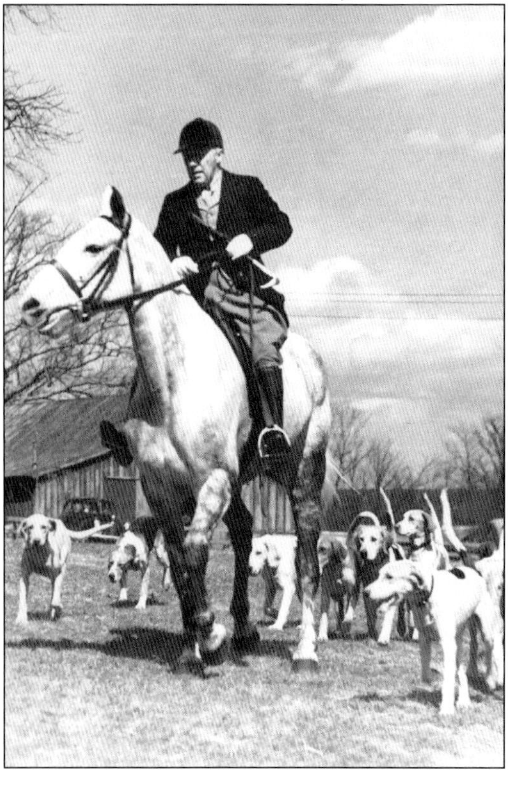

In 1940, Margaret Lindsley Warden, seen here at the front left, joined several other Nashvillians as the "Valient" took its first drive at its winter home. Coaching became a popular sport for the ultra-rich in the late 1800s, and it has continued to be an elite equestrian activity. (Courtesy of Gore Center.)

Mason Houghland, Master of Fox Hounds, founded the Hillsboro Hounds in 1932. Here he leads out the pack before a foxhunt in the 1940s or 1950s. Houghland published his nationally acclaimed book about foxhunting, *Gone Away*, in 1949, thus establishing the Hillsboro Hounds and Middle Tennessee as leaders in American foxhunting. (Courtesy of Gore Center.)

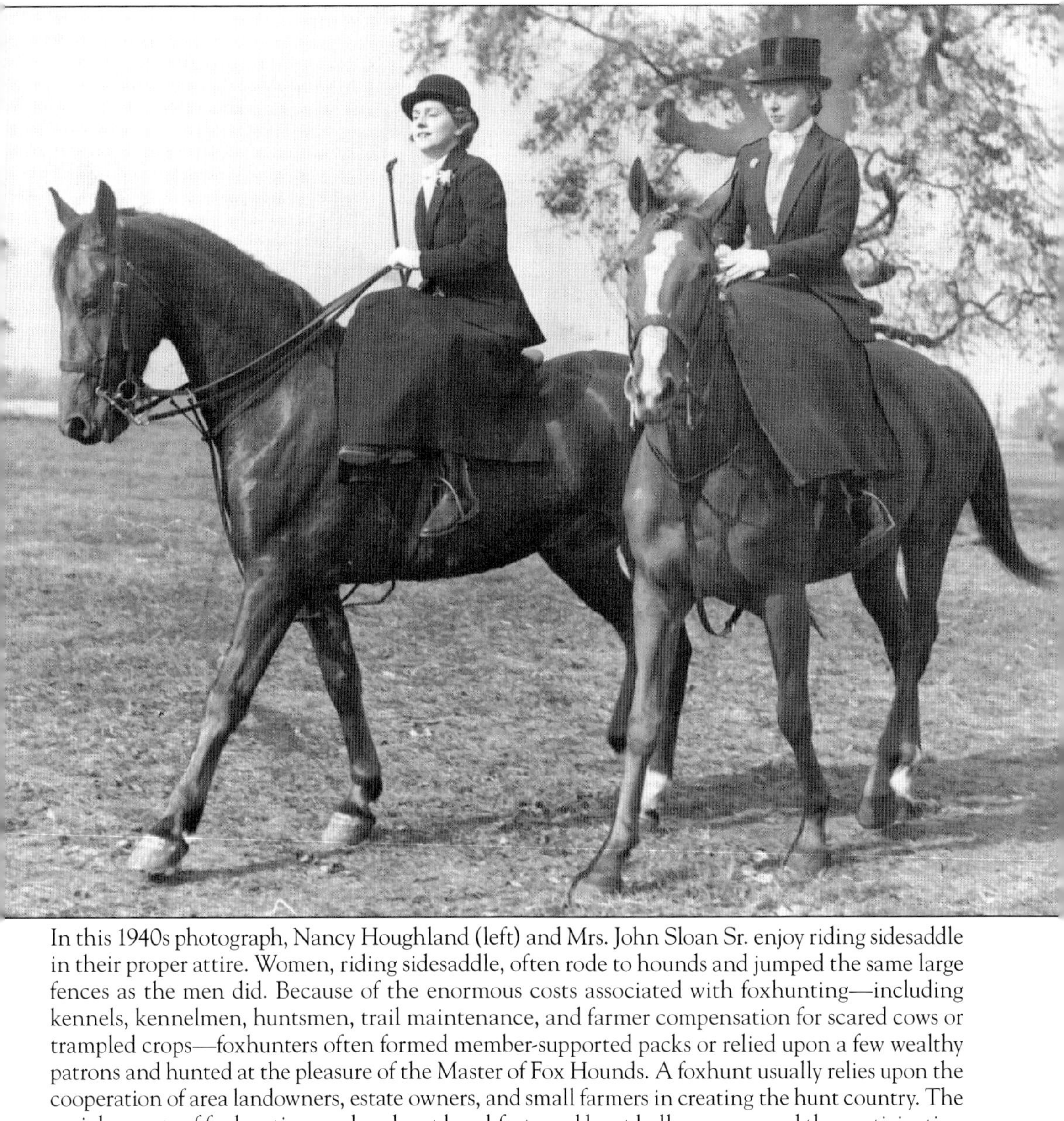

In this 1940s photograph, Nancy Houghland (left) and Mrs. John Sloan Sr. enjoy riding sidesaddle in their proper attire. Women, riding sidesaddle, often rode to hounds and jumped the same large fences as the men did. Because of the enormous costs associated with foxhunting—including kennels, kennelmen, huntsmen, trail maintenance, and farmer compensation for scared cows or trampled crops—foxhunters often formed member-supported packs or relied upon a few wealthy patrons and hunted at the pleasure of the Master of Fox Hounds. A foxhunt usually relies upon the cooperation of area landowners, estate owners, and small farmers in creating the hunt country. The social aspects of foxhunting, such as hunt breakfasts and hunt balls, encouraged the participation of both sexes. After World War II, foxhunting clubhouses slowly turned into golf and country clubs. The Sloans and Houghlands had led the development of Brentwood (incorporated in 1969) as an equestrian-oriented community in the 1930s and 1940s. (Courtesy of Gore Center.)

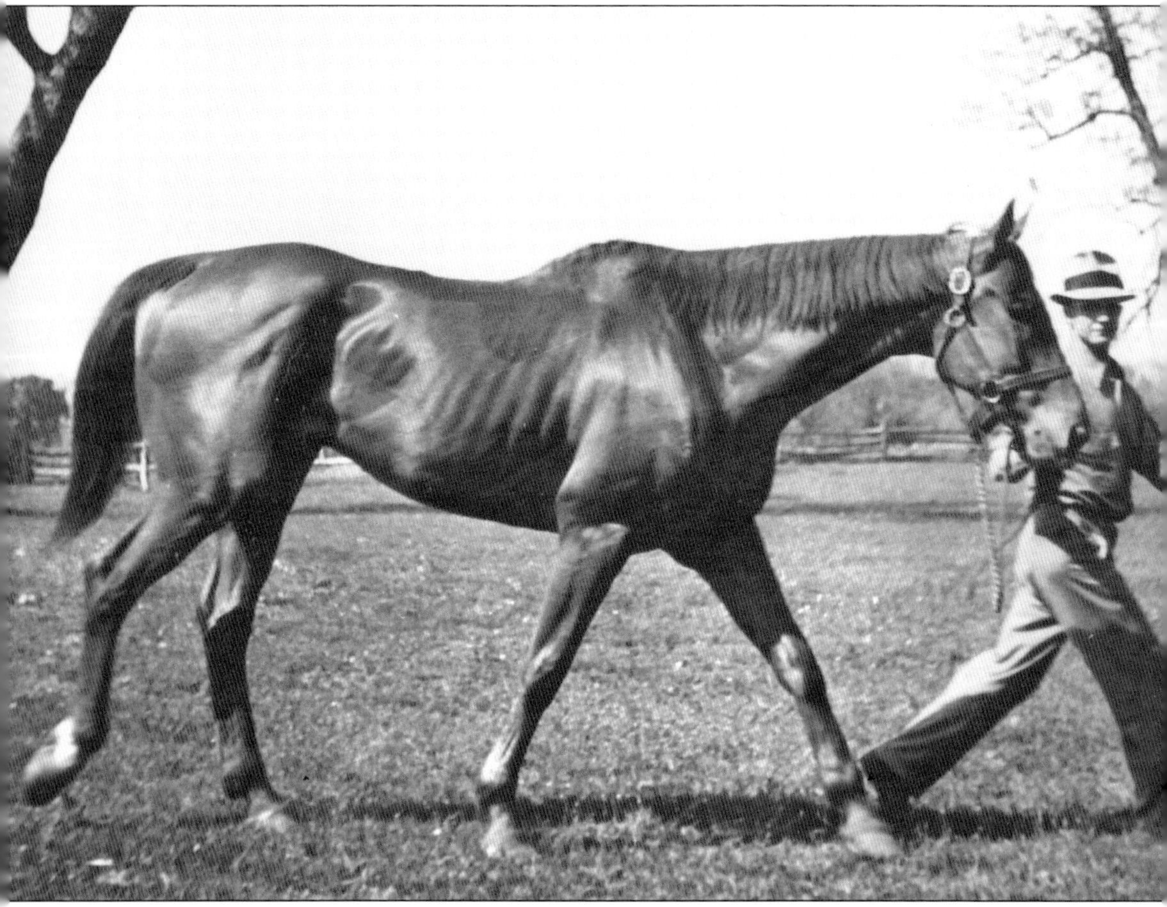

Bryon Hilliard of Louisville, Kentucky, leads his Thoroughbred Big Bird before winning the 1933 running of the Tennessee Timber Toppers steeplechase at Overton Downs in Nashville. Steeplechasing originated in England in 1792, but it did not become an organized sport in the United States until the late 1890s. In 1895, a group of foxhunters, concerned horse owners and trainers, and racetrack owners joined to form the Hunt Race and Steeplechase Association. Foxhunters, often the mainstays of local steeplechases, usually became involved in steeplechasing when they realized that a particular hunt horse could gallop faster or jump higher than the rest of the field could. During the 1920s and 1930s, steeplechasing took place in at least two other locations in Middle Tennessee: There was a track in Smyrna, and another was located at Grasslands (the former Fairview plantation) in Gallatin. William DuPont, a leading Thoroughbred breeder and racehorse owner, designed the Iroquois course. Its annual race is held on the second Saturday in May. (Courtesy of Gore Center.)

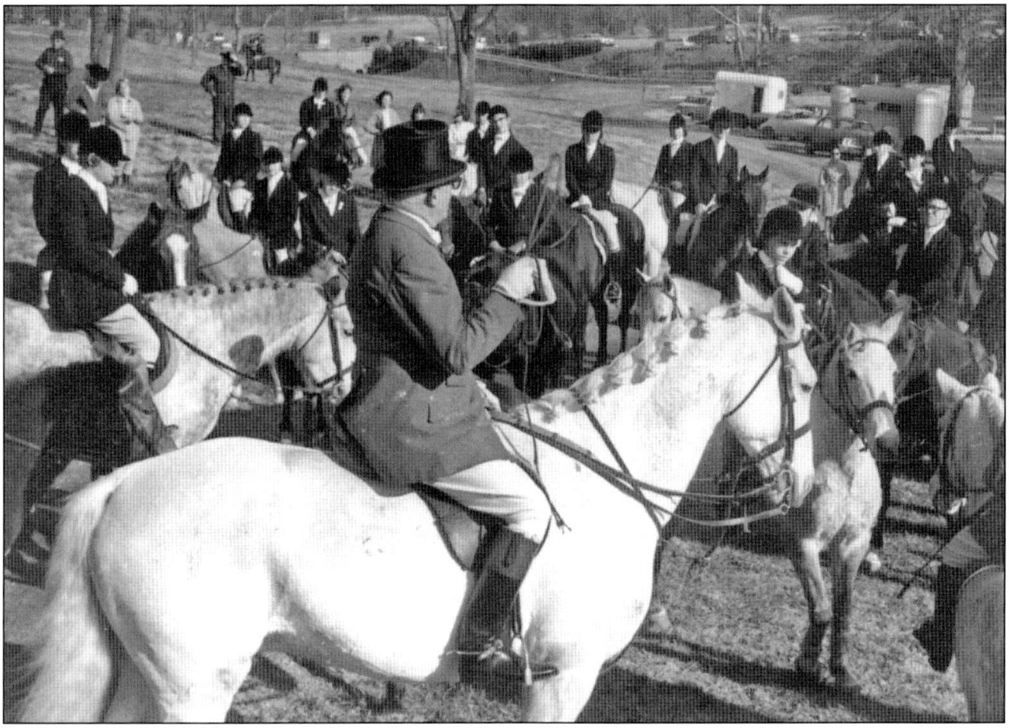

This 1966 Middle Tennessee Pony Club, gathering at Henry W. Hooker's with the Hillsboro Hounds, provided an opportunity for children to participate in foxhunting. These sponsored hunts, arranged by invitation only, were many pony clubbers' only foxhunting experiences. Hooker published his foxhunting memoir, *Fox, Fin, and Feather*, in 2001. The books highlights Middle Tennessee's sporting life. (Courtesy of Gore Center.)

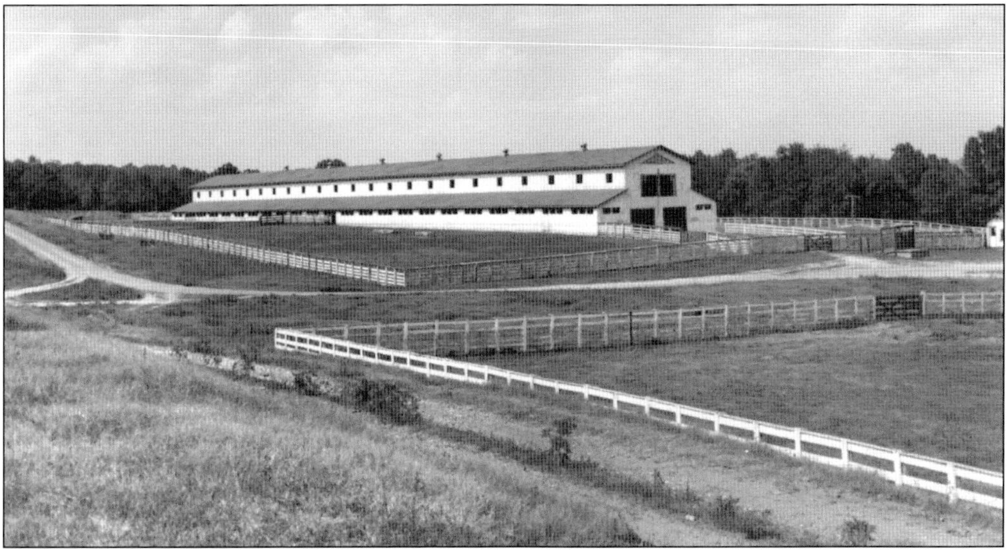

This view of the stable at Milky Way Farm introduces another set of important Middle Tennessee Thoroughbred breeders. From 1931 to 1933, Franklin and Ethel Mars, the candy manufacturers, designed and built this estate near Pulaski as a racehorse nursery and training facility. The farm produced the 1940 Kentucky Derby winner Galladion. (Courtesy of TSLA.)

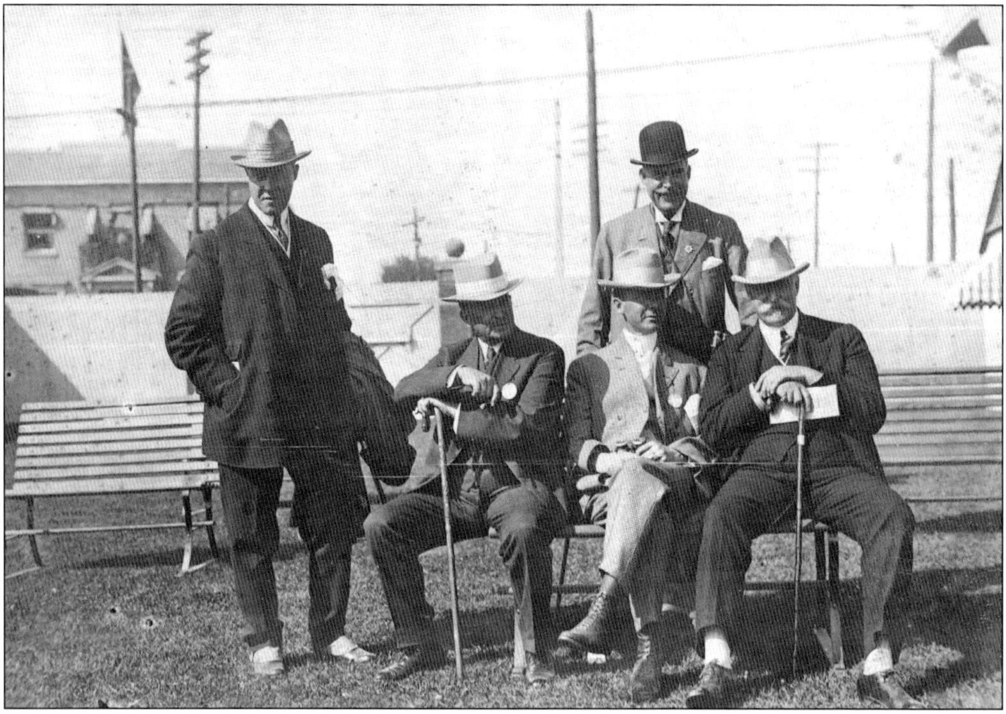

Walter O. Parmer (right) is accompanied by four unidentified men at a Nashville area racecourse in the first decade of the 1900s. A prominent Thoroughbred breeder, Parmer established his farm, Edenwold Stud, in 1903 on land that once belonged to Belle Meade. He began his breeding program with one of Belle Meade's former stallions, the Commoner. (Courtesy of Gore Center.)

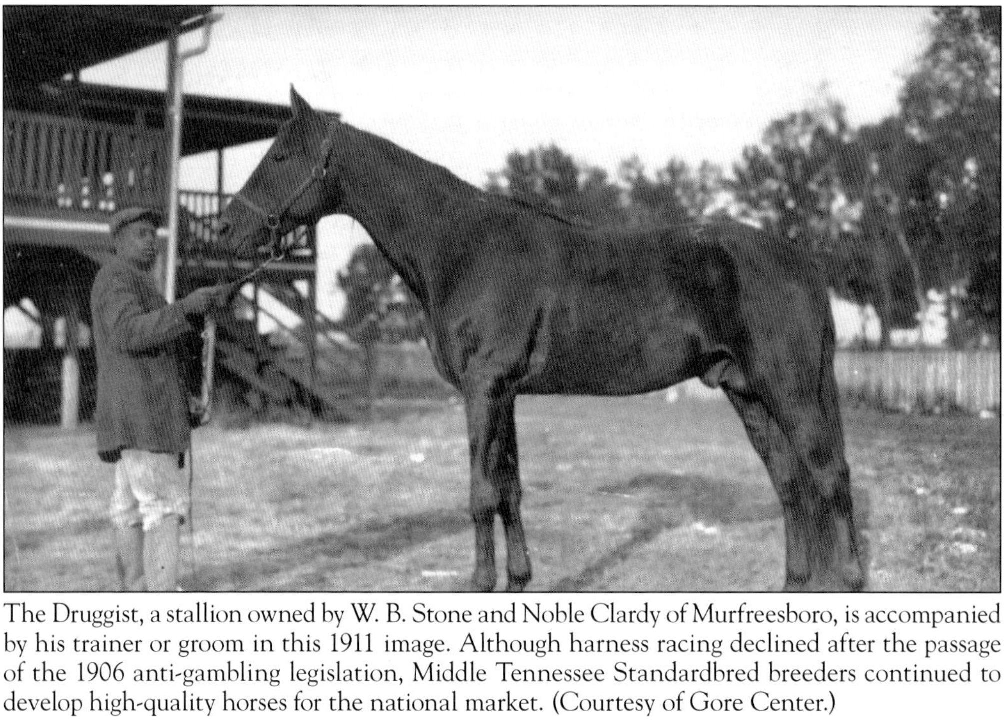

The Druggist, a stallion owned by W. B. Stone and Noble Clardy of Murfreesboro, is accompanied by his trainer or groom in this 1911 image. Although harness racing declined after the passage of the 1906 anti-gambling legislation, Middle Tennessee Standardbred breeders continued to develop high-quality horses for the national market. (Courtesy of Gore Center.)

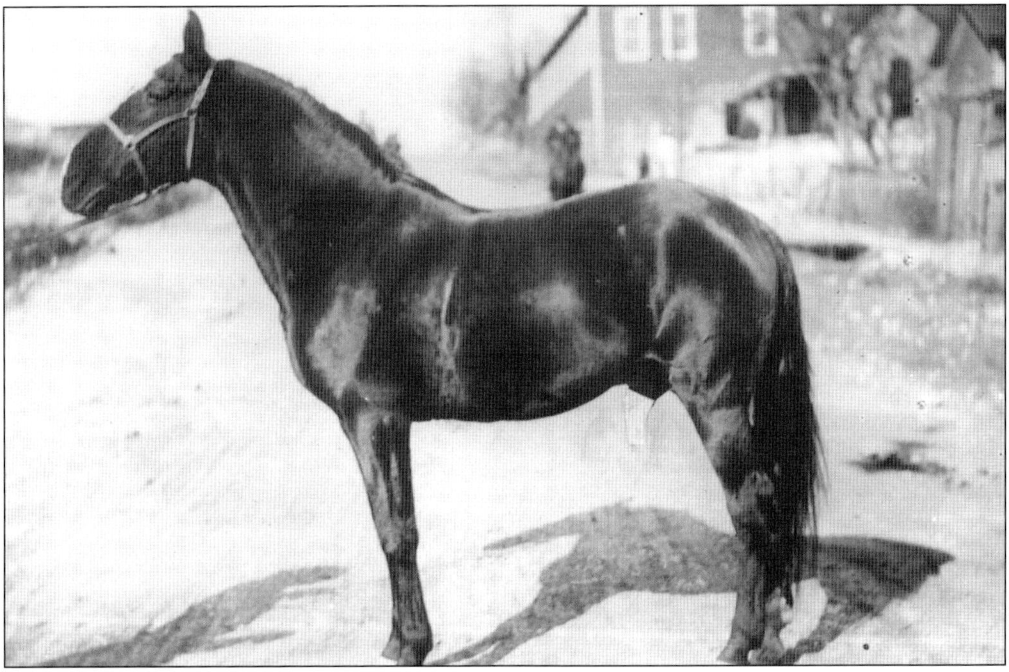

The pacer Walter Direct, whose one-mile record was 2:05.74, was owned by the Chaffin Brothers Company of Columbia. The stallion was most likely photographed at South Side Park, a racetrack and training facility leased by the Chaffin brothers from the Tennessee Fair Association. The brothers reportedly turned down an offer of $12,500 for this horse. (Courtesy of Gore Center.)

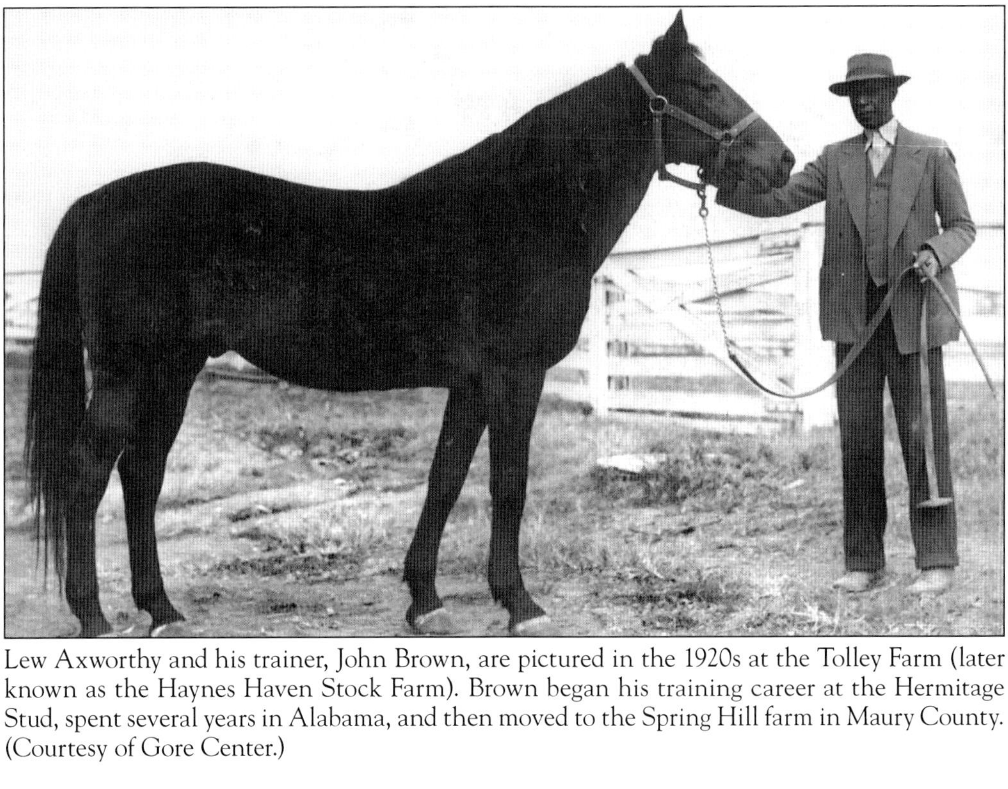

Lew Axworthy and his trainer, John Brown, are pictured in the 1920s at the Tolley Farm (later known as the Haynes Haven Stock Farm). Brown began his training career at the Hermitage Stud, spent several years in Alabama, and then moved to the Spring Hill farm in Maury County. (Courtesy of Gore Center.)

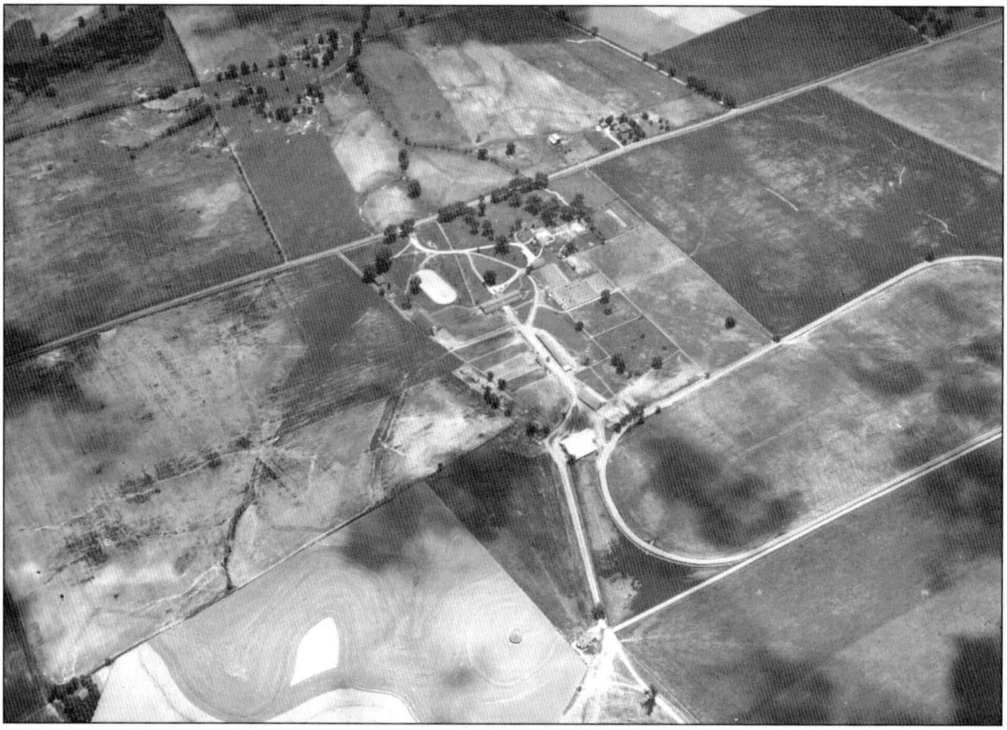

This 4,000-foot aerial view of Haynes Haven, photographed in May 1940 by the Tennessee Department of Conservation, shows the track used to train the Tolley Farm's Standardbreds. Tolley Farm became a Tennessee Walking Horse farm, Haynes Haven, in 1939 and was the home of Haynes Peacock, the Grand Champion in 1940 and 1941. (Courtesy of TSLA.)

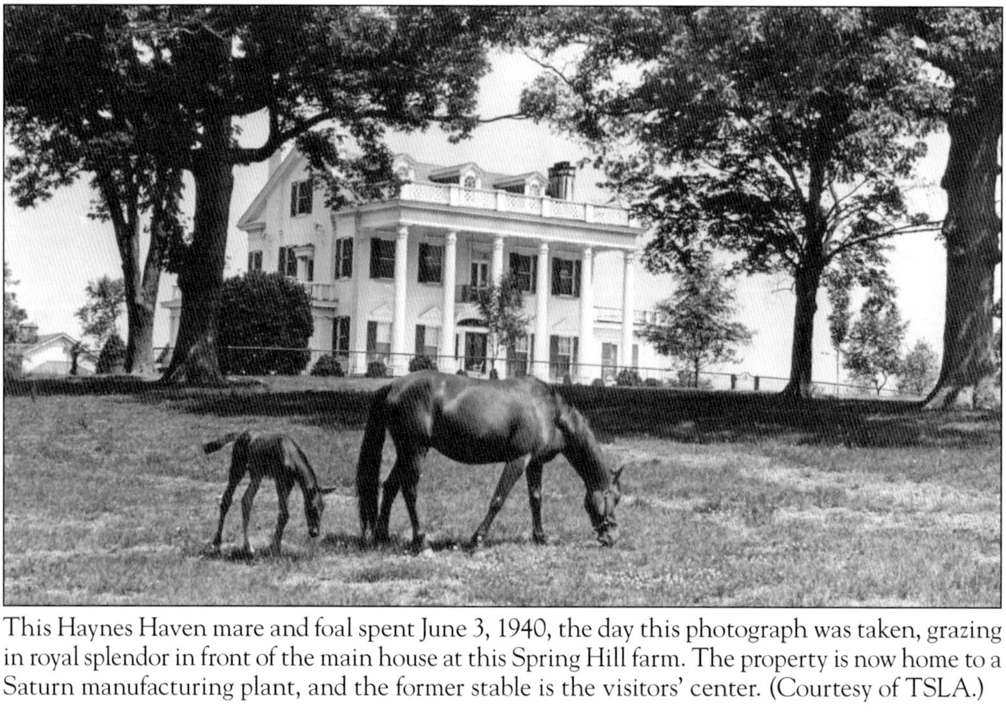

This Haynes Haven mare and foal spent June 3, 1940, the day this photograph was taken, grazing in royal splendor in front of the main house at this Spring Hill farm. The property is now home to a Saturn manufacturing plant, and the former stable is the visitors' center. (Courtesy of TSLA.)

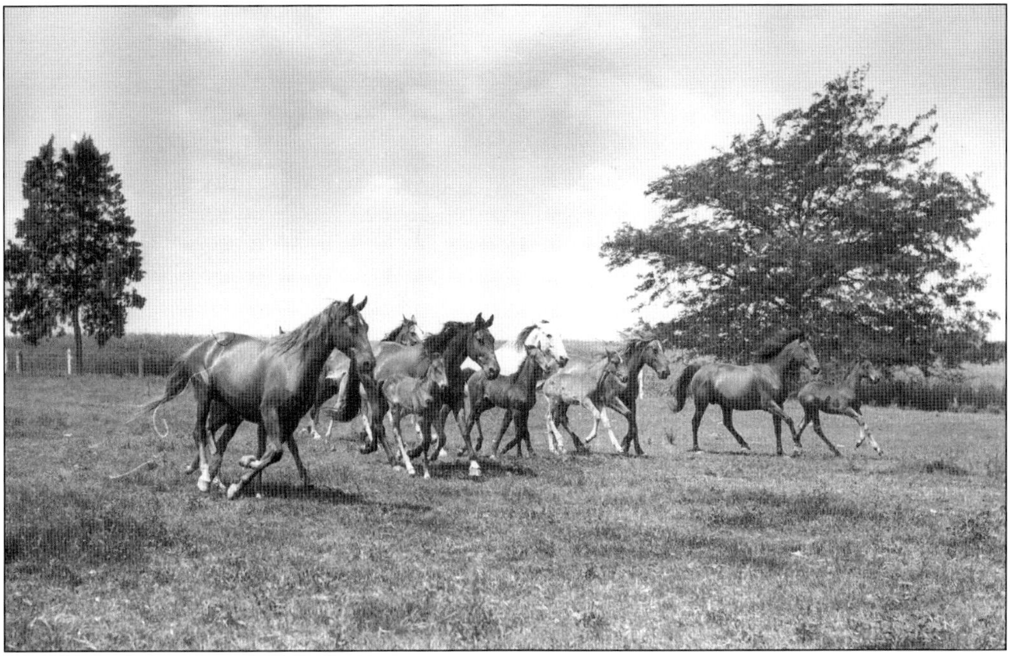

These mares and foals cantering through the pasture at Haynes Haven on May 30, 1940, exemplify the resurgence of horse breeding in Middle Tennessee by the early 1940s. Breeders were willing to invest in large pieces of property in order to provide enough grazing land for their young horses. (Courtesy of TSLA.)

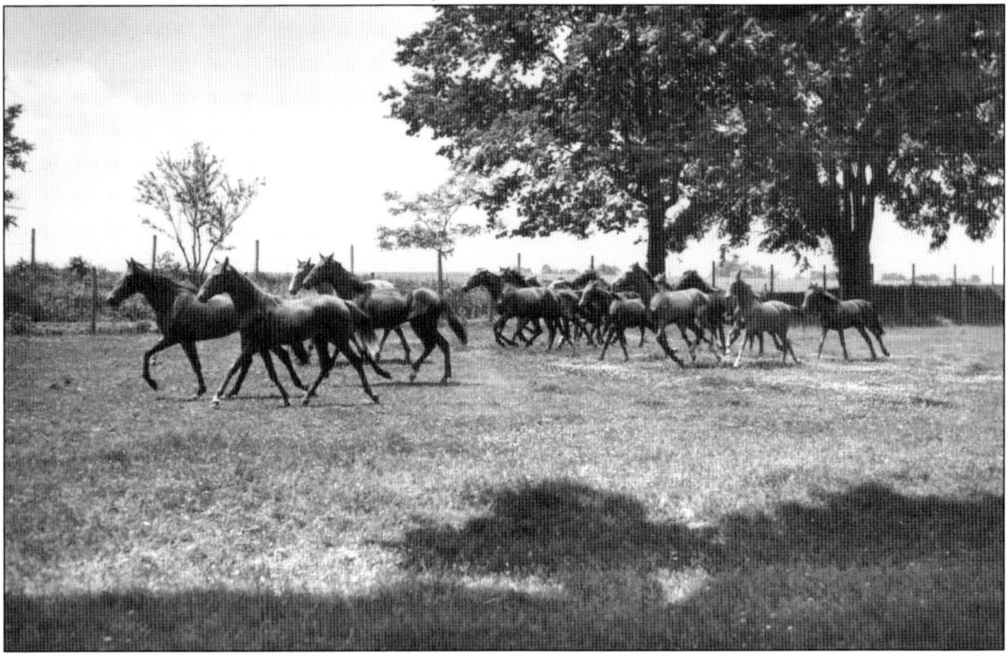

These Haynes Haven yearlings trot through their pasture in Spring Hill on May 30, 1940. The Tennessee Department of Conservation took these photographs to convey the importance of the Tennessee Walking Horses—and of all horses—in Middle Tennessee's agricultural and economic development. (Courtesy of TSLA.)

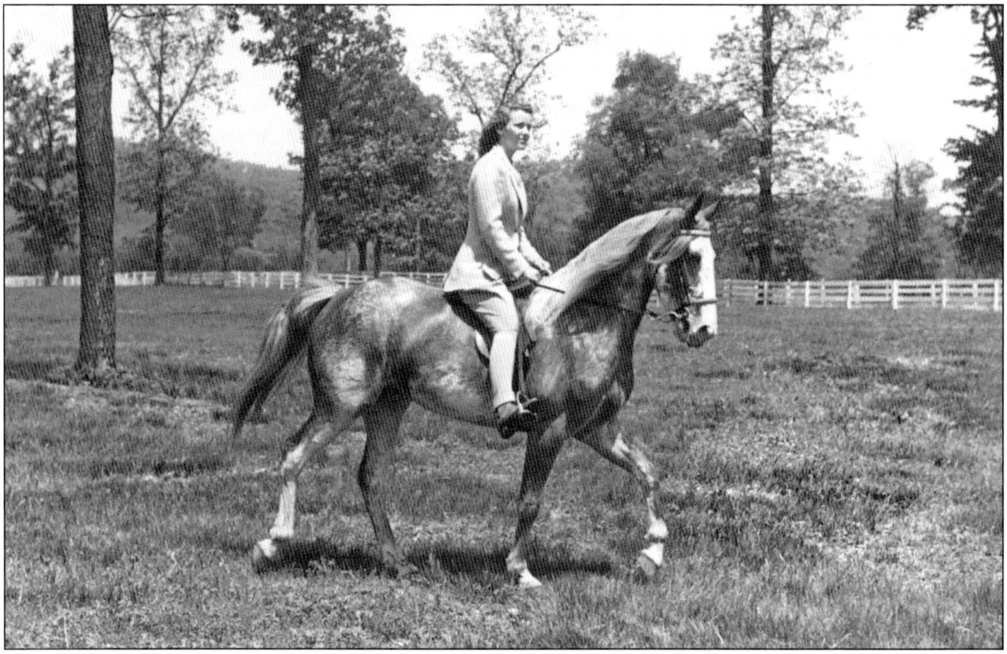

This Maryland Farm Saddlebred demonstrates the breed's characteristic movement while being ridden by Ethel Devine on April 30, 1941. Two years later, Earl Teater, a leading trainer from Harrodsburg, Kentucky, joined Maryland Farm as its trainer, directing further national attention toward Middle Tennessee and toward Brentwood in particular. (Courtesy of TSLA.)

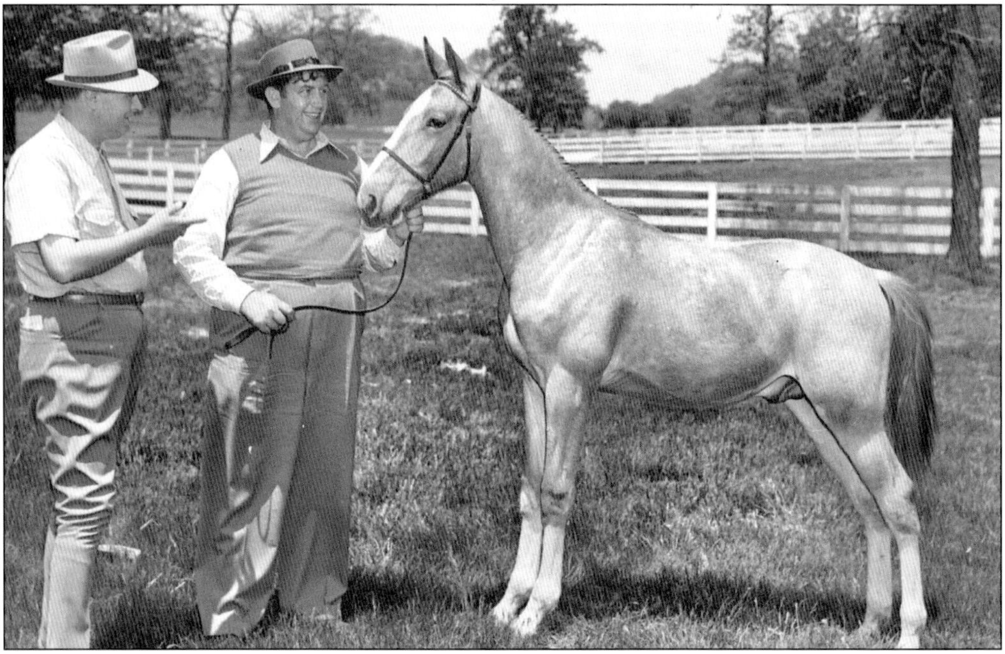

J. Truman Ward (left) and Andy Devine stand with a Standardbred on April 30, 1941. The Devines' April 1940 trip to Maryland Farm was a media event combining the best of Middle Tennessee's high-quality horses and hospitality. In 1974, Maryland Farms became the site of a major office complex. (Courtesy of TSLA.)

Six

KIDS AND PONIES

Although Middle Tennessee children have been riding horses, ponies, donkeys, and mules since the first settlers arrived in the region, it was not until the late 19th century that parents began to acquire mounts specifically for their children. American society as a whole had begun to treat children as young people, rather than as miniature adults. The Middle Tennessee youngsters highlighted in this chapter illustrate their families' willingness to spend time and money on their children's equestrian activities. Some of these families earned their livings as horse breeders and trainers, but most were upper- and middle-class families whose participation in horse sports helped to establish their identities within Middle Tennessee society.

Until 1953, most Middle Tennessee children had to compete in the "12 and under" classes at the local fairs, charity horse shows, and festivals. Margaret Lindsley Warden changed that in 1953, when she convinced the Williamson County Horseman's Association to sponsor a competition for public and private school students. After a coordinated campaign of parental requests, editorials in Warden's "Horse Sense" column, and promised sponsorships from local businesses, the Williamson County School Board acquiesced, and the Interschool Riding Tournament began.

Between its inaugural event in 1953 and the final competition in 1974, the Interschool Riding Tournament gave "horsey" kids of all backgrounds the opportunity to represent their schools. Teams included four or five students, who often used monogrammed saddle pads or wore armbands with the school's initials. Students participated in gymkhana, jumping, western, and saddle seat events that encouraged a wide range of skill levels and types of mounts. The competition was widely popular throughout Middle Tennessee. Some of the participating schools included Central High (Fayetteville), Donelson, Ensworth, Lipscomb, Franklin High, Gower, Grassland, Harpeth Hall, Hillsboro, Hillwood, Overton Intermediate, Peabody, Percy Priest, Robertson Academy, St. Cecilia, St. Henry, and Two Rivers.

Warden's second accomplishment in 1953 was the establishment of the Middle Tennessee Pony Club (MTPC). The next year, the MTPC became one of the U.S. Pony Clubs' five charter members. Today the MTPC remains a leader in the U.S. Pony Clubs' Mid-South region and continues to produce nationally ranked members.

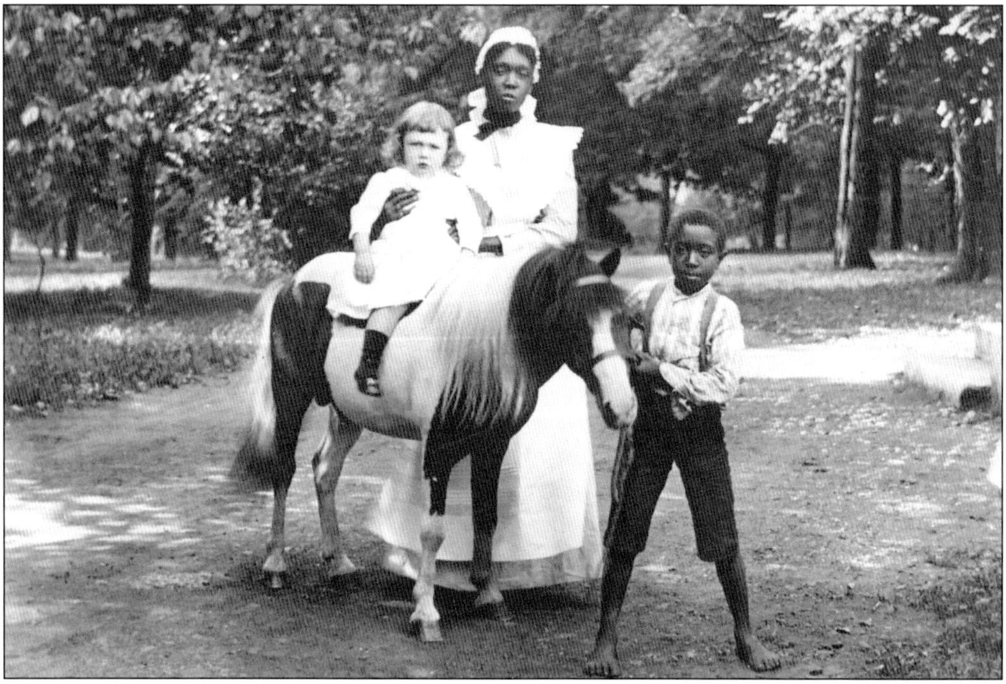

William H. Jackson Jr., heir to the Belle Meade Plantation, rides one of the family's ponies in the late 1890s. Along with other purebred livestock, the family raised English Shetland ponies. The boy is accompanied by his nursemaid and a stable boy. (Courtesy of TSLA.)

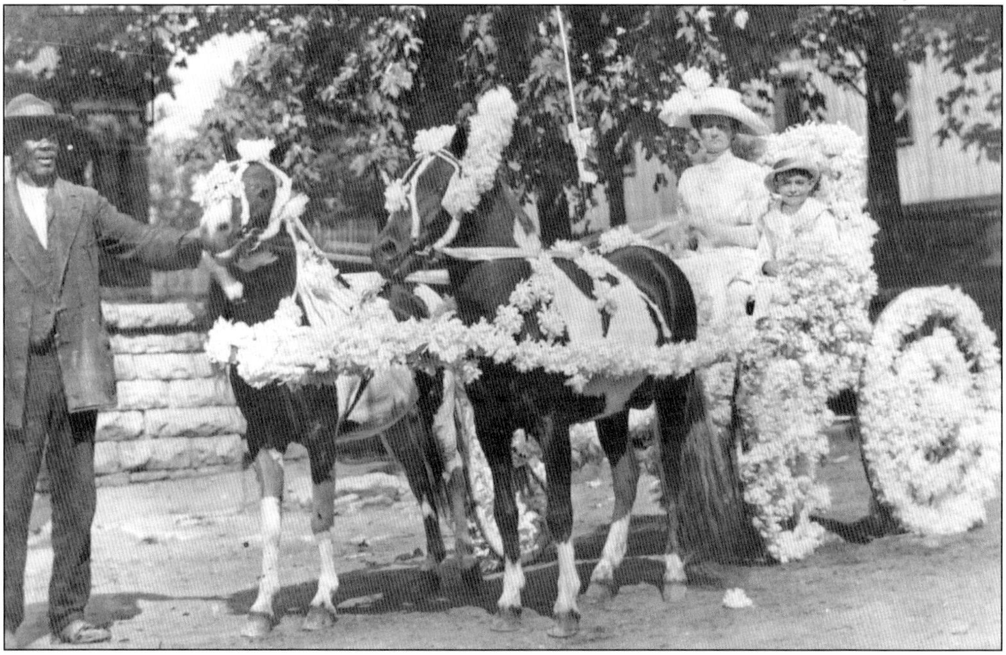

The unidentified woman and boy in this flower-bestrewn carriage were almost certainly participants in one of the numerous annual parades that were held in towns throughout Middle Tennessee. Late-19th-century children were exposed to the thrills of horse sports through their participation in public events such as this one, which took place in the 1880s. (Courtesy of Gore Center.)

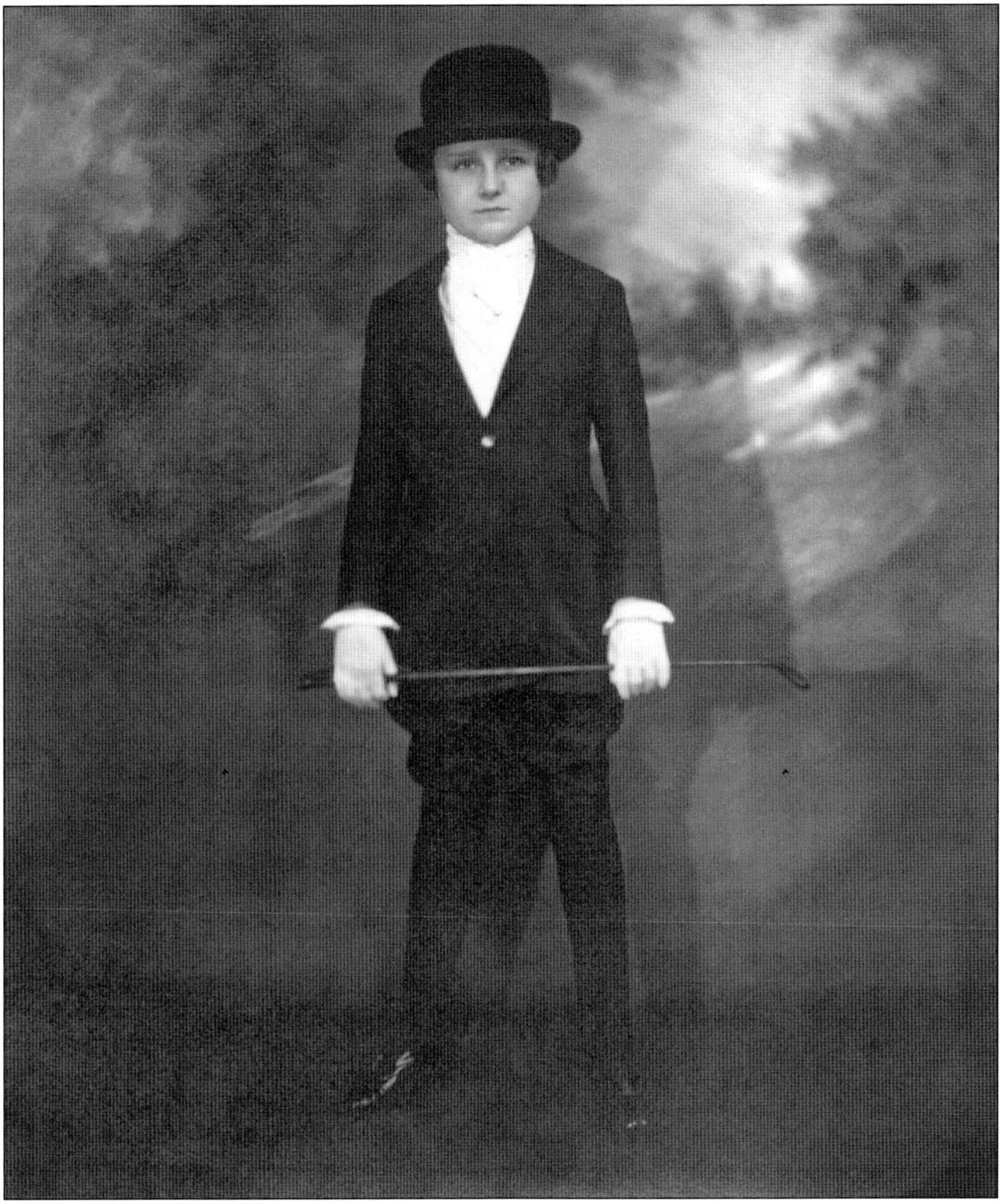

Shirley Caldwell Patterson shows off the proper saddle-seat attire of a young Nashvillian of the 1920s in this studio photograph. The proper clothing, tack, and horse needed for a child to be able to compete in the show ring or ride in the hunt field could be costly. Children usually wear the same types of clothing as adults. In this photograph, Patterson wears a bowler cap, a white stock tie with a gold pin, a black show coat with tails, flared black britches, and patent leather paddock boots. The safety helmet, commonly seen on children today, was not developed until the early 1980s. Riding helmets have evolved more in the last 20 years than they did in the previous 200. Although the styles of the clothing have changed slightly, the basic materials and cuts have remained the same. (Courtesy of Gore Center.)

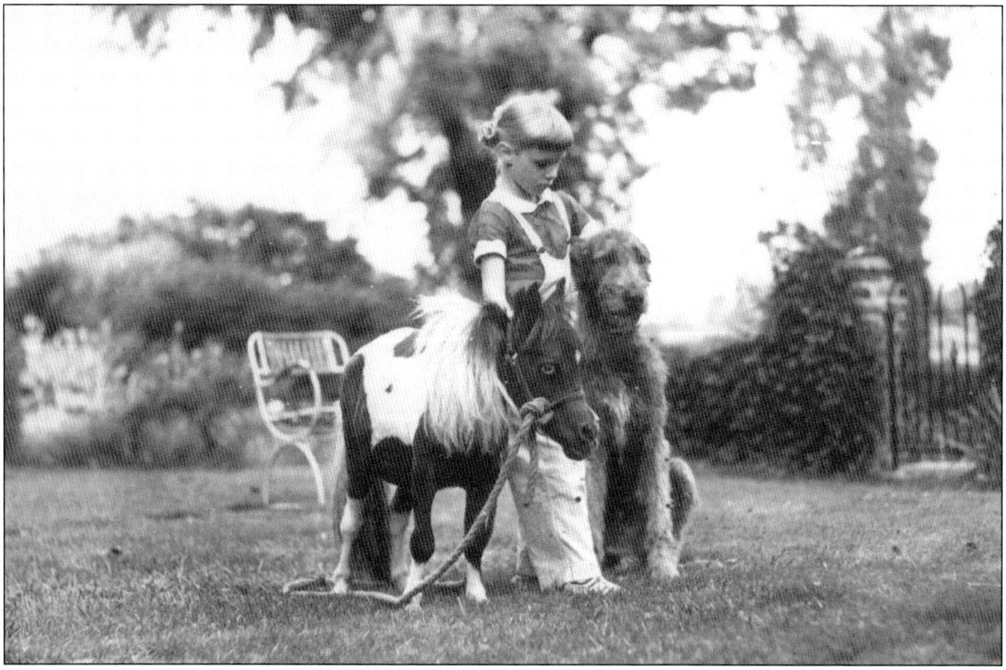

Above, Maxie Dickinson, a daughter of Jacob McGavock Dickinson, stands in the garden at Travellers Rest in the early 1930s, accompanied by a miniature horse and a large hunting dog. Maxie and her siblings, all of whom rode the family's Arabian horses, were the last descendants of Travellers Rest founder John Overton. Below, Maxie Dickinson and several of her friends play with model horses in front the Dickinson children's play barn in the 1930s. The children also had a three-room Gothic Revival playhouse, as well as other places for their amusement, on the rural farm. (Above courtesy of Gore Center; below courtesy of Travellers Rest Plantation and Museum.)

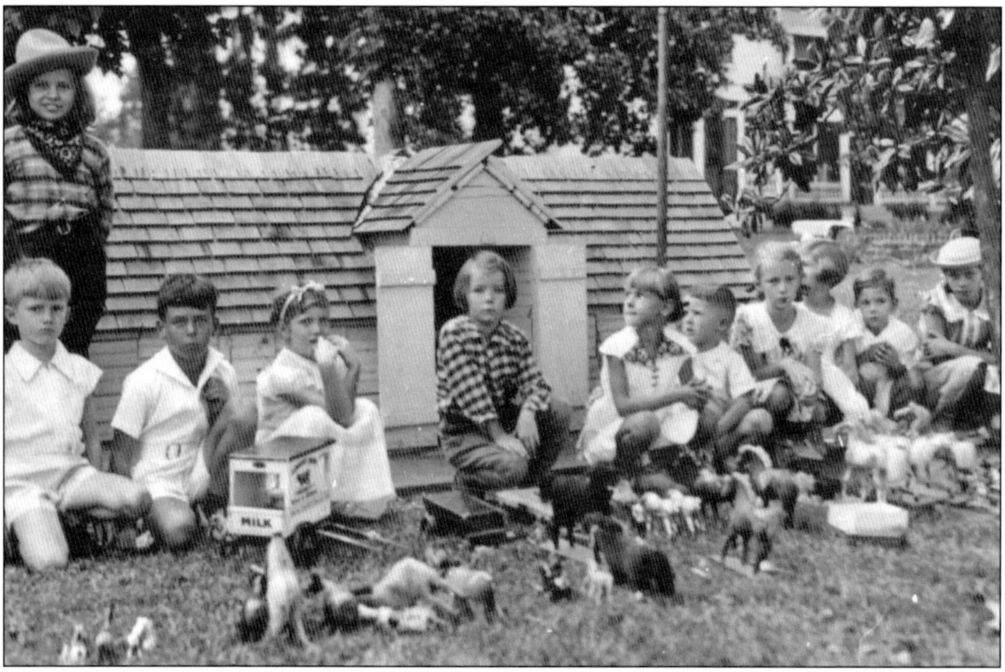

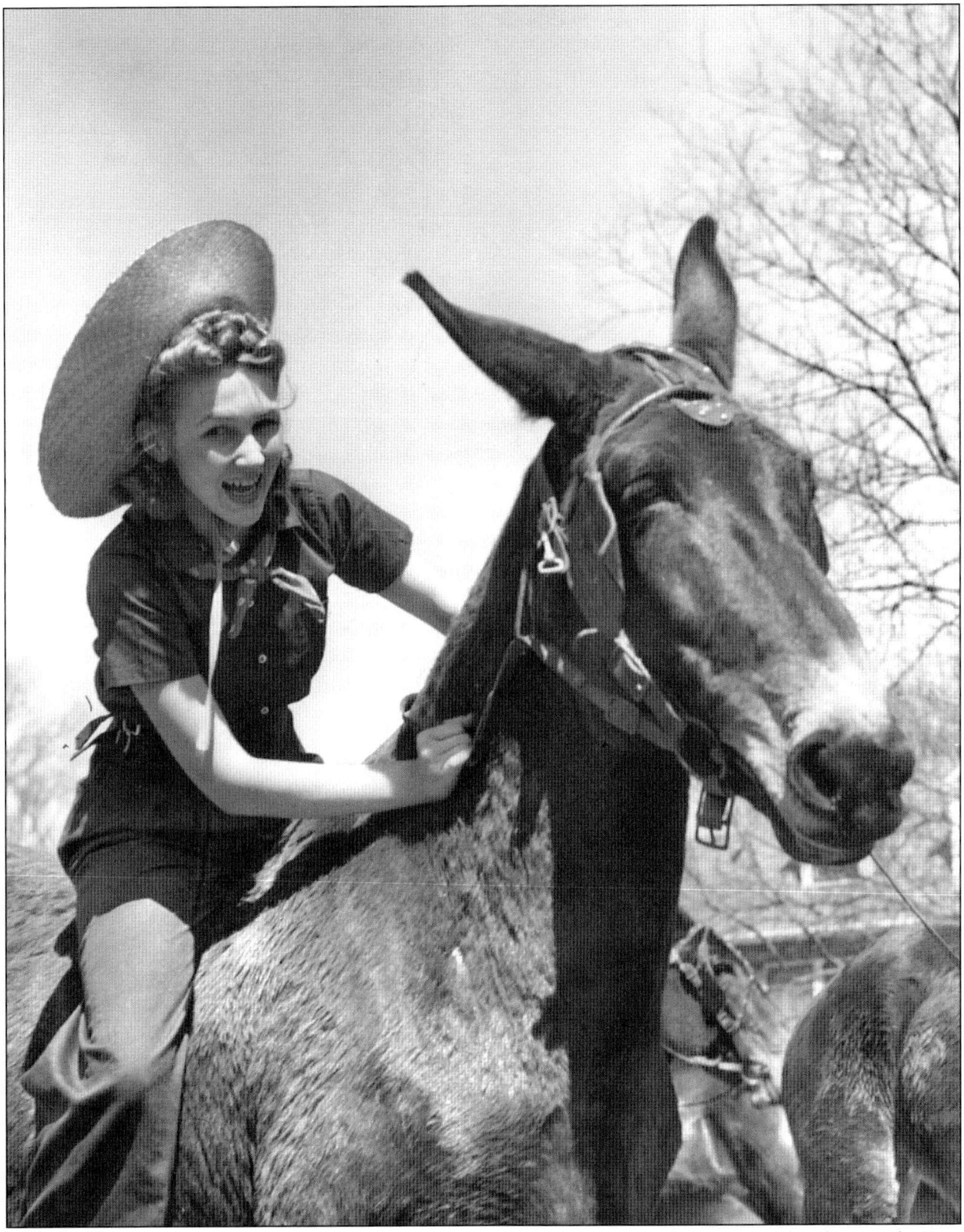

Lucille Keith of Maury County shows off for the camera during the 1939 Columbia Mule Day parade. Her mount is one of the famous Middle Tennessee mules. One of the parade's early advertising slogans was "1,000 girls on a 1,000 mules." In some years, it was not false advertising. The mule's quiet nature and sensibility almost certainly enabled more than one child or timid rider the opportunity to participate in one of Middle Tennessee's premier cultural events. In the last decade, the parade has regularly attracted over 100,000 participants and spectators. (Courtesy of TSLA.)

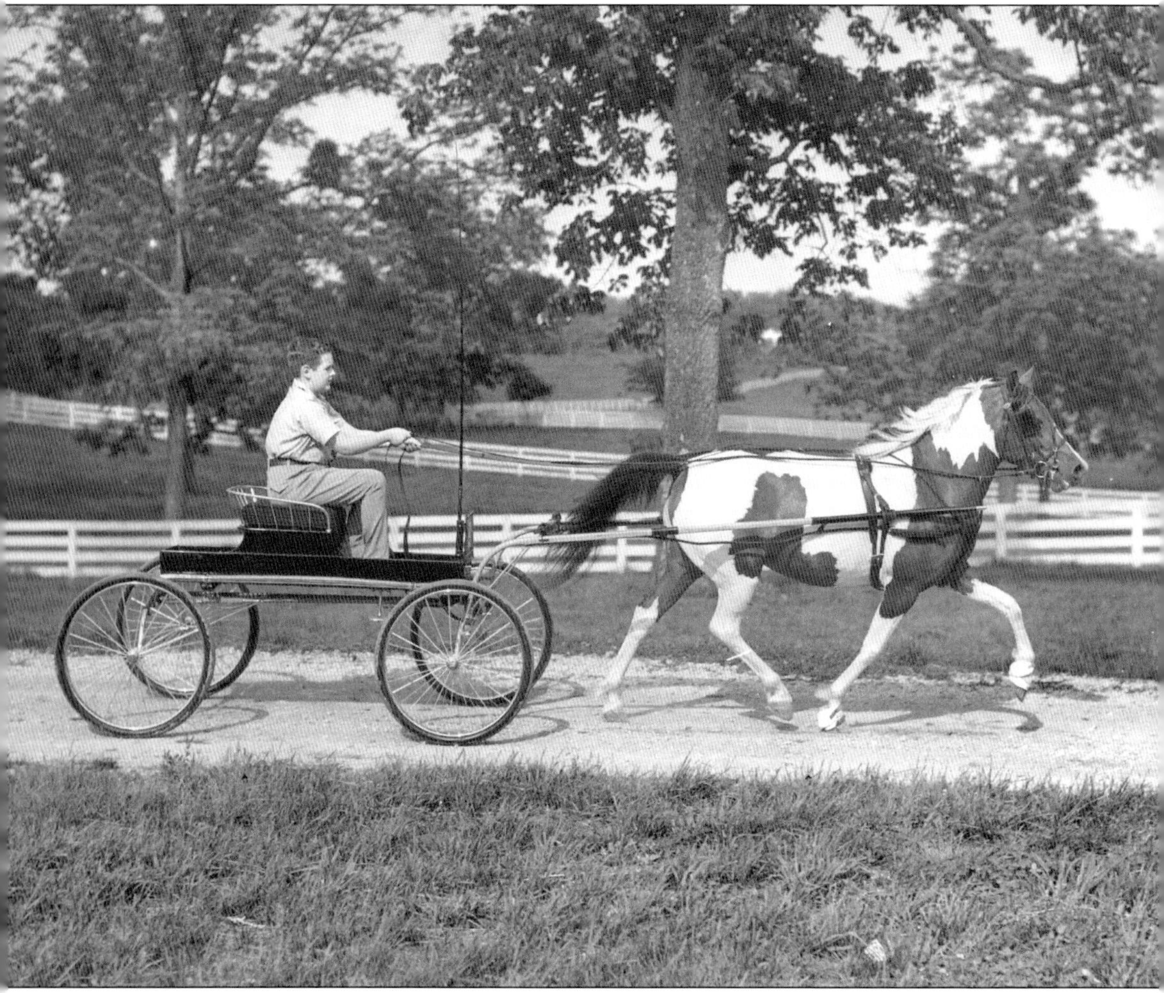

Jimmy Ward, son of Maryland Farm owner J. Truman Ward, drives his gaited pony across the Brentwood breeding farm in May 1940. Driving a cart at any speed takes coordination, but driving a cart for the show ring, as Ward did, requires skill and quick reactions. Although the family primarily showed its breeding stock as a marketing tool, it is reasonable to assume that Jimmy Ward also attended some of the American Saddlebred shows. The entry would have been judged on the pony's movement and way of going and on Ward's ability to handle the cart in an enclosed arena. (Courtesy of TSLA.)

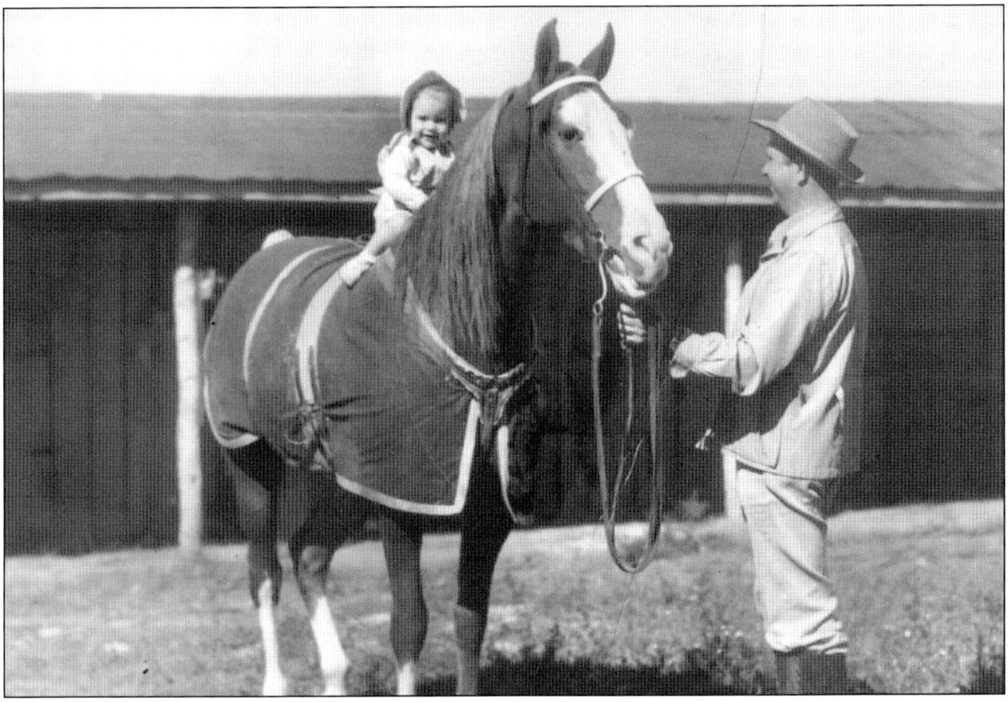

Tennessee Walking Horse trainer Winston Wiser holds Merry Gypsy Rose as his daughter, Judy Wiser, sits on top of the blanketed mare. Wiser trained three horses to five Grand Championships at the Tennessee Walking Horse National Celebration, including two-time champion Merry Go Boy, a half-brother to Merry Gypsy Rose. (Courtesy of Gore Center.)

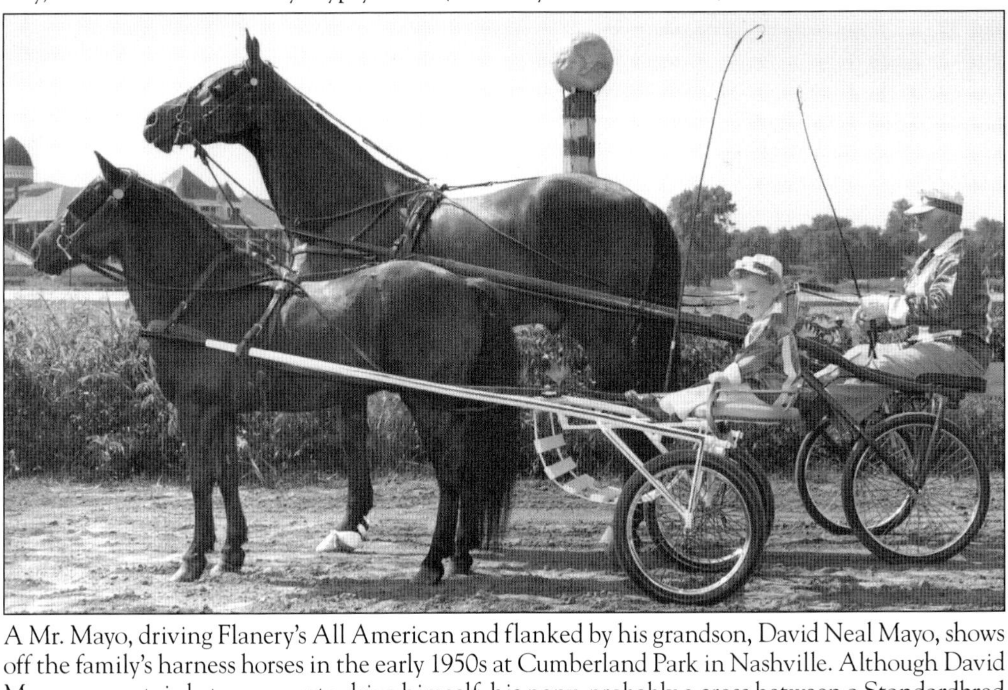

A Mr. Mayo, driving Flanery's All American and flanked by his grandson, David Neal Mayo, shows off the family's harness horses in the early 1950s at Cumberland Park in Nashville. Although David Mayo was certainly too young to drive himself, his pony, probably a cross between a Standardbred and a pony or smaller horse, is ready for the task. (Courtesy of Gore Center.)

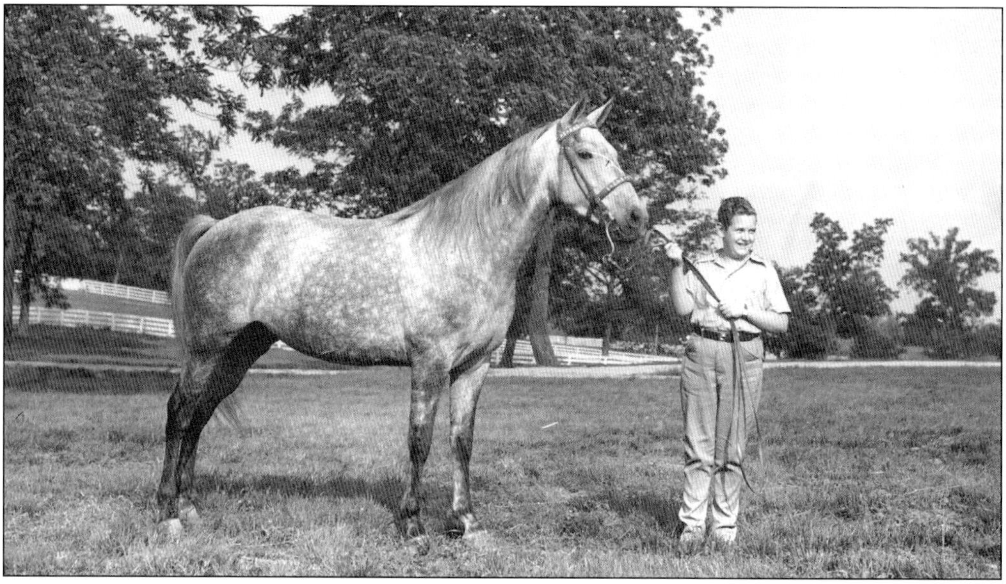

Jimmy Ward was about 12 years old when this photograph was taken at Maryland Farm in May 1940. Although many 1940s children from the cities and new suburban areas never got the ponies they dreamed of, Ward was able to experience life with horses throughout the year, fulfilling his desires for four-legged companionship. (Courtesy of TSLA.)

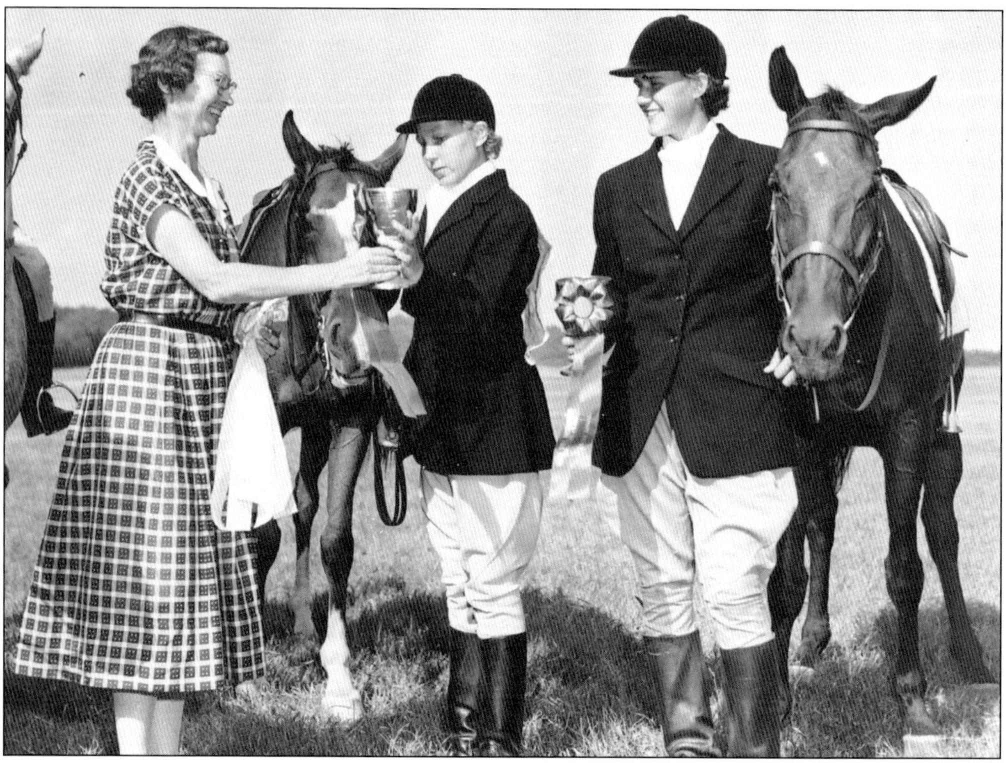

In this 1955 photograph at the Horse Sense Tournament, Margaret Lindsley Warden is handing an award to Judy Kinnard with her horse Tidewater, as Kernan Regen and her horse Royal Bug watch. Both of these girls were members of the Mid-South Pony Club. (Courtesy of Gore Center.)

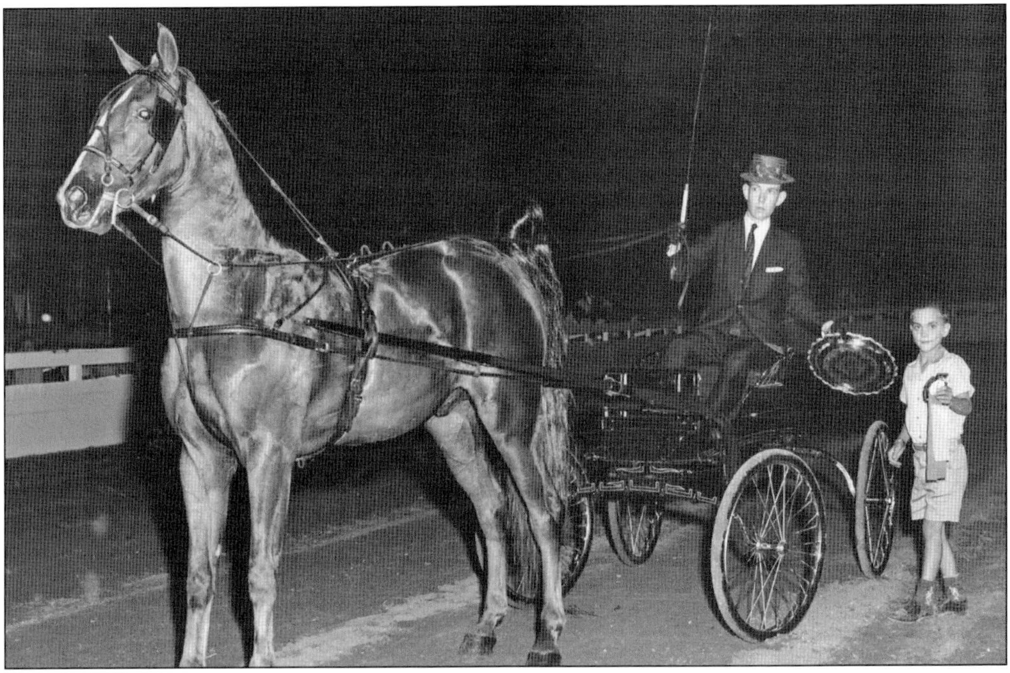

This 1950s competitor and his horse Citizen Cain, from Brown View Farm in Murfreesboro, are receiving a ribbon. Although there were (and still are) fewer boys than girls at the adolescent levels throughout the horse industry, the percentages became more equal at the professional level. (Courtesy of Nashville Public Library, the Nashville Room.)

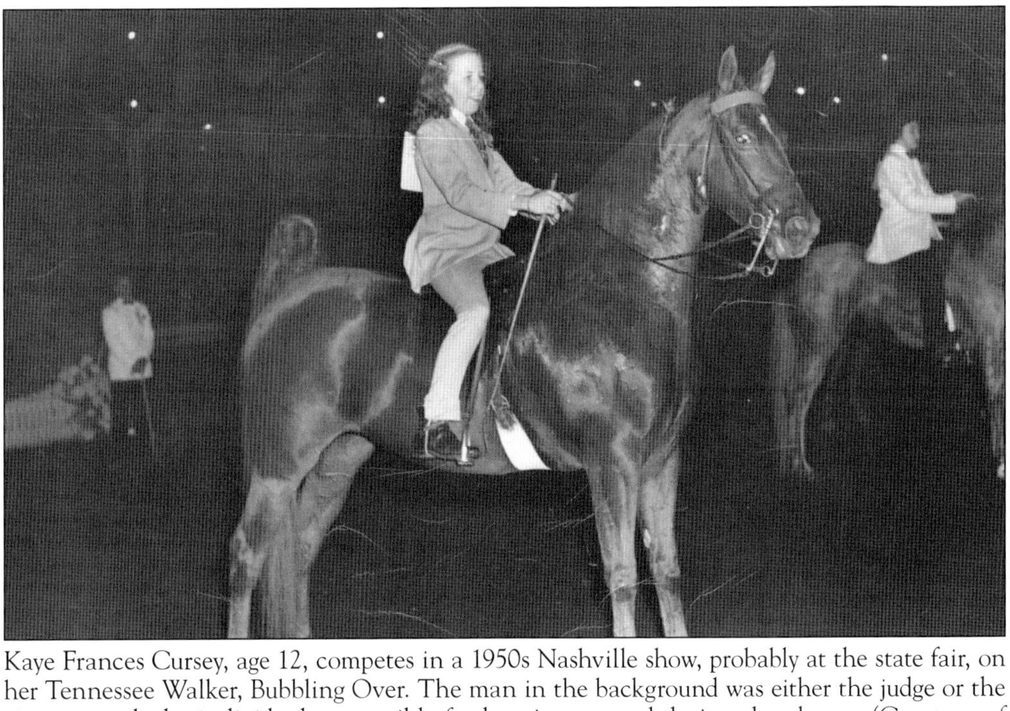

Kaye Frances Cursey, age 12, competes in a 1950s Nashville show, probably at the state fair, on her Tennessee Walker, Bubbling Over. The man in the background was either the judge or the ring steward, the individual responsible for keeping control during the classes. (Courtesy of Gore Center.)

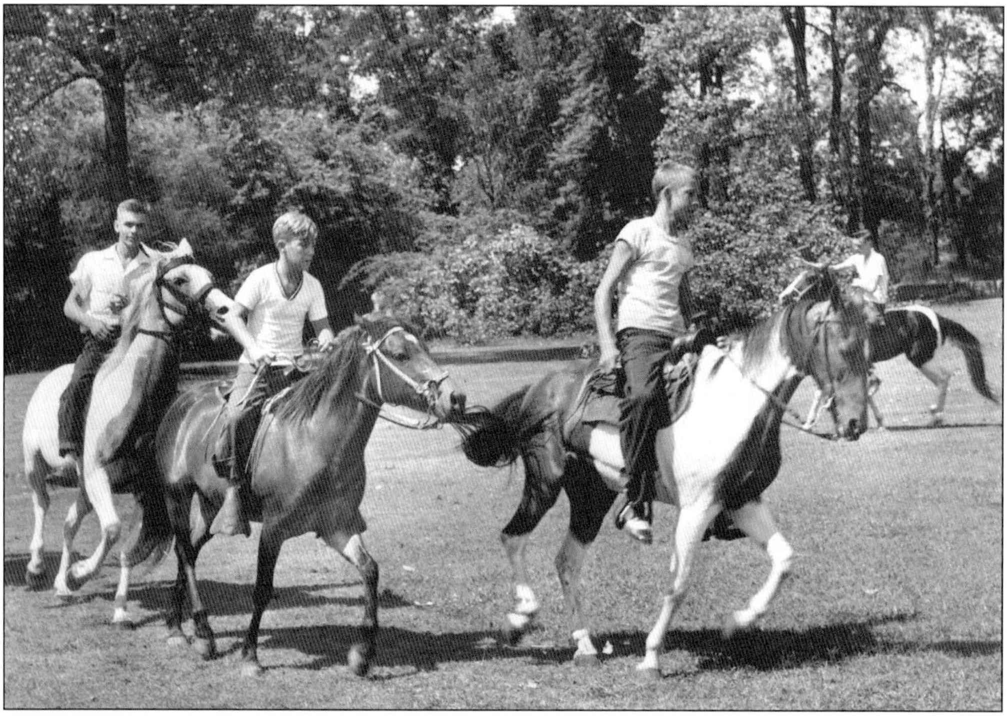

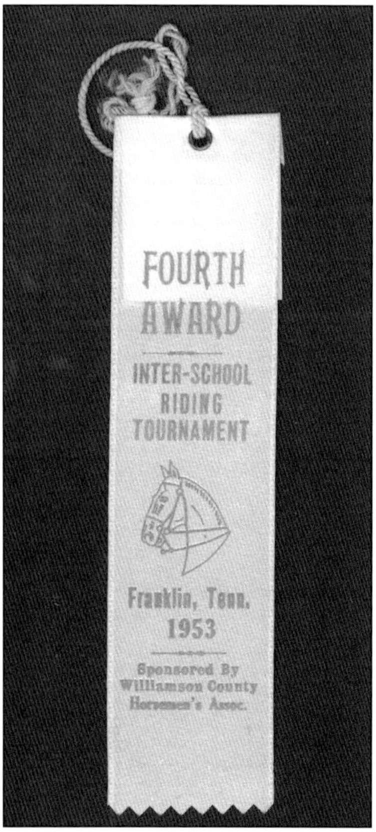
FOURTH
AWARD
INTER-SCHOOL
RIDING
TOURNAMENT
Franklin, Tenn.
1953
Sponsored By
Williamson County
Horsemen's Assoc.

Seen here from left to right, Johnny Burroughs, Johnny Merriman, and Billy Nane participate in a mid-1950s western drill team pattern at a local horse show. Many mid-20th-century shows were sponsored by local benevolent organizations, such as the Elks or Lions Clubs, to raise funds for their charitable work. (Courtesy of Gore Center.)

This fourth-place ribbon is a physical reminder of Margaret Lindsley Warden's efforts to create a series of shows for Middle Tennessee schoolchildren. Within a few years of the inaugural competition of the Interschool Riding Tournament in 1953, several of the participating schools began holding team trials and practice sessions because of the tournament's popularity. (Courtesy of Gore Center.)

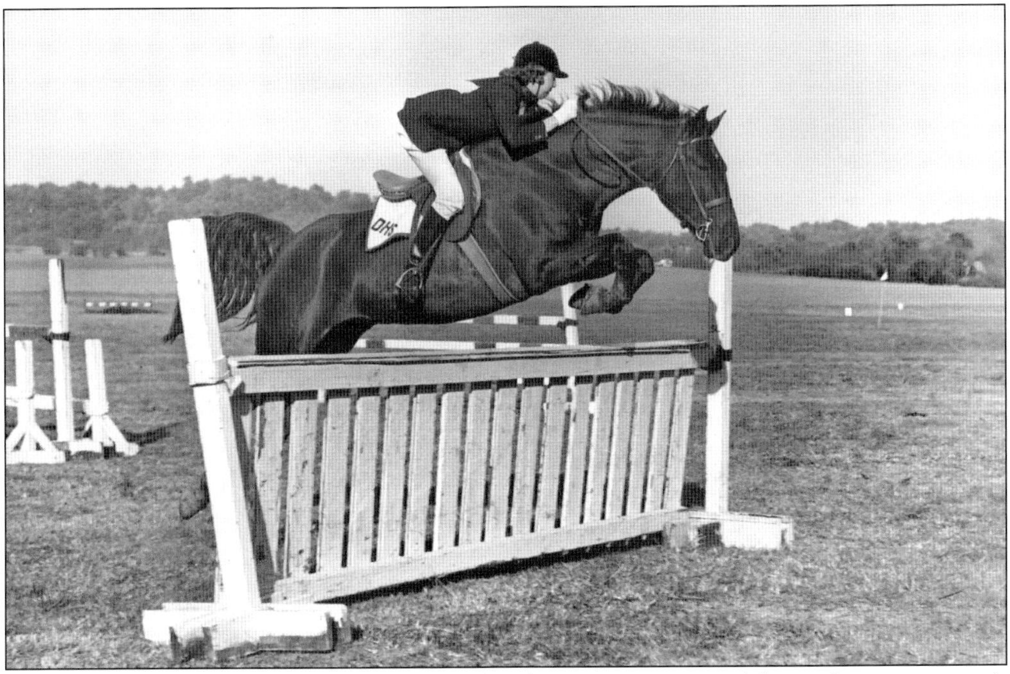

These two images from the 1962 Interschool Riding Tournament celebrate the competition's 10th anniversary. Many of the children participating that year had older siblings who had ridden during the 1950s, making the competition a family tradition. Several children who successfully competed in regular shows also joined these school teams. Above, Donelson's senior team member Jane Card and her mount easily clear a large gate in a stadium course set up on the grounds of Percy Warner Park in Nashville. Below, Gower's intermediate team prepares for competition in the western riding events. (Courtesy of Gore Center; photographs by Iroquois of Nashville.)

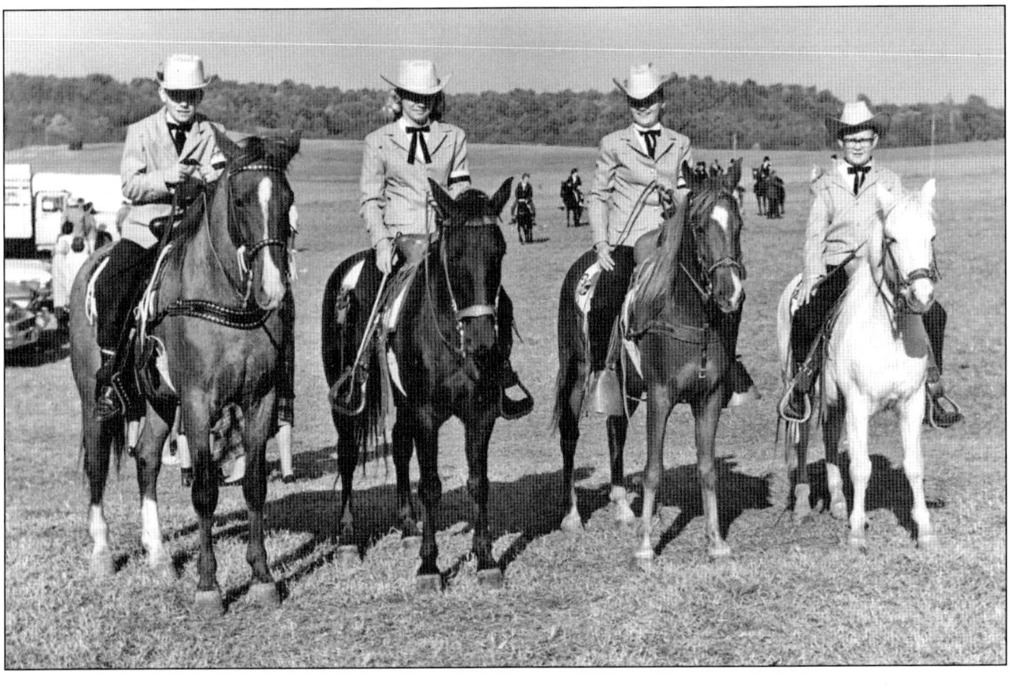

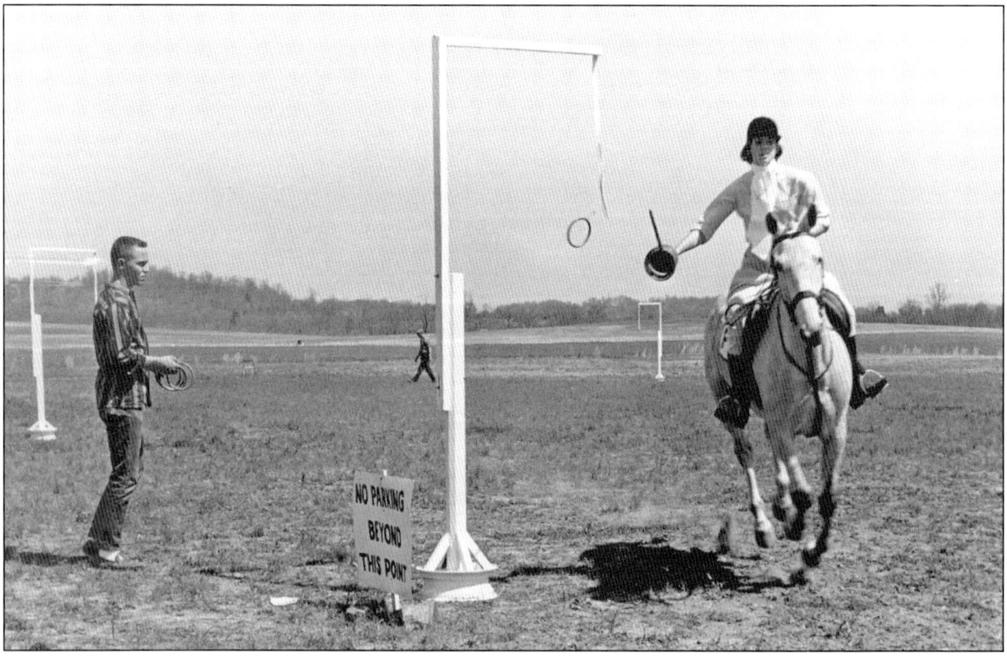

This rider is competing in the ring race at the Interschool Riding Tournament on March 30, 1963. Gymkhana events, first popularized in Great Britain by the British Pony Club, began to grow in popularity in the postwar era. These races test a rider and horse's skill and precision, rather than athletic ability or beauty. (Courtesy of Gore Center; photograph by Iroquois of Nashville.)

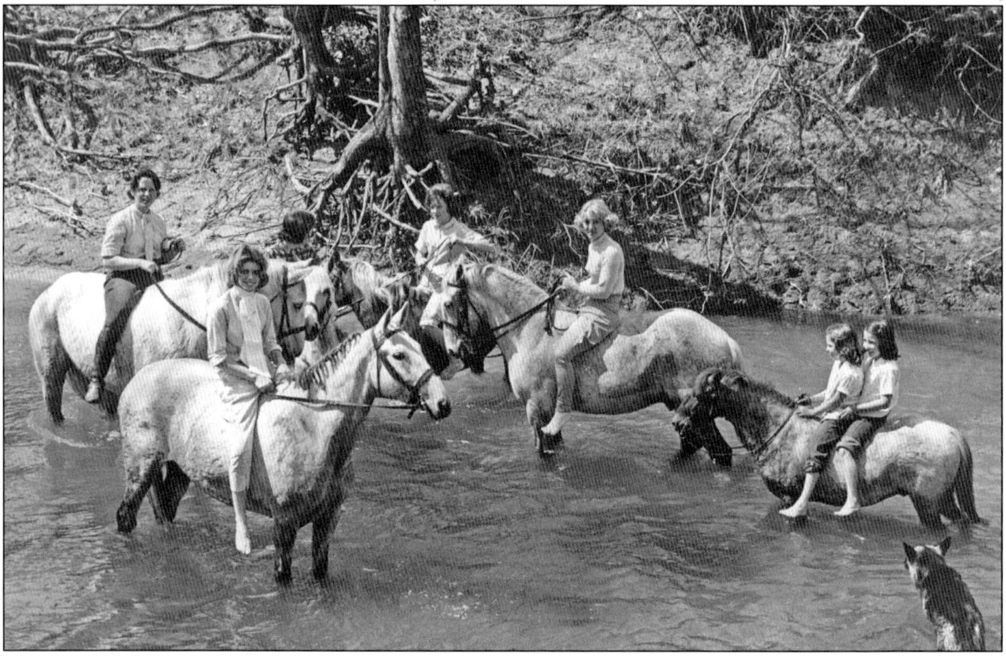

These six horses, seven kids, and one dog found the Harpeth River after the conclusion of the 1963 Interschool Riding Tournament. Their obvious pleasure makes it clear why many Middle Tennessee parents wholeheartedly embraced the "horsey" world as an opportunity for recreation and social interaction for their children. (Courtesy of Gore Center; photograph by Iroquois of Nashville.)

Seven

1945–2005

In the late 1940s, as Middle Tennesseans returned to lives free from rationing and saving, they used their accumulated resources to resume breeding and riding their horses. These two generations of horse enthusiasts continued to build upon the region's heritage of horse breeding while also expanding its breadth and depth. The American Quarter Horse, a relatively new breed considering the dates of the establishment of pedigree registers, made rapid inroads into Middle Tennessee, and western riding, popularized by the stars of Western movies, became common. The Tennessee Walking Horse industry underwent some adjustments in its rules and standards, but the enthusiasm for the horse continued unabated. The three other older breeds—Thoroughbreds, Standardbreds, and Saddlebreds—also had similar setbacks and advances.

The sports that increased the most during these six decades are those that fall into the "forward riding" category, as Margaret Lindsley Warden described them in a November 26, 1956, "Horse Sense" review of Capt. Vladimir S. Littauer's seminal book *Schooling Your Horse*. Warden was an ardent promoter of correct (balanced) riding of any form, but especially of the international events of dressage (training), show jumping, and eventing. She used her position at the *Tennessean* to invite the German dressage trainer Erich Bubbel to Nashville for a dressage clinic in March 1954. It was the first public demonstration of dressage in Middle Tennessee.

On Labor Day weekend in 1954, Middle Tennessee welcomed the nation's top three-day event riders, including Maj. Jonathan R. Burton, J. E. B. Wofford, Walter Staley Jr., and many multi-starred generals (who had overseen the military teams) to the country's first Olympic three-day trial that was open to civilians. In 2004, the Middle Tennessee Horse Trials celebrated its 50th anniversary.

Dressage, hunter, and jumper trainers and breeders have developed important breeding and training facilities in Middle Tennessee, especially in the corridor from Murfreesboro to Franklin, where horses of all breeds have won national and international championships in grand prix dressage and show jumping.

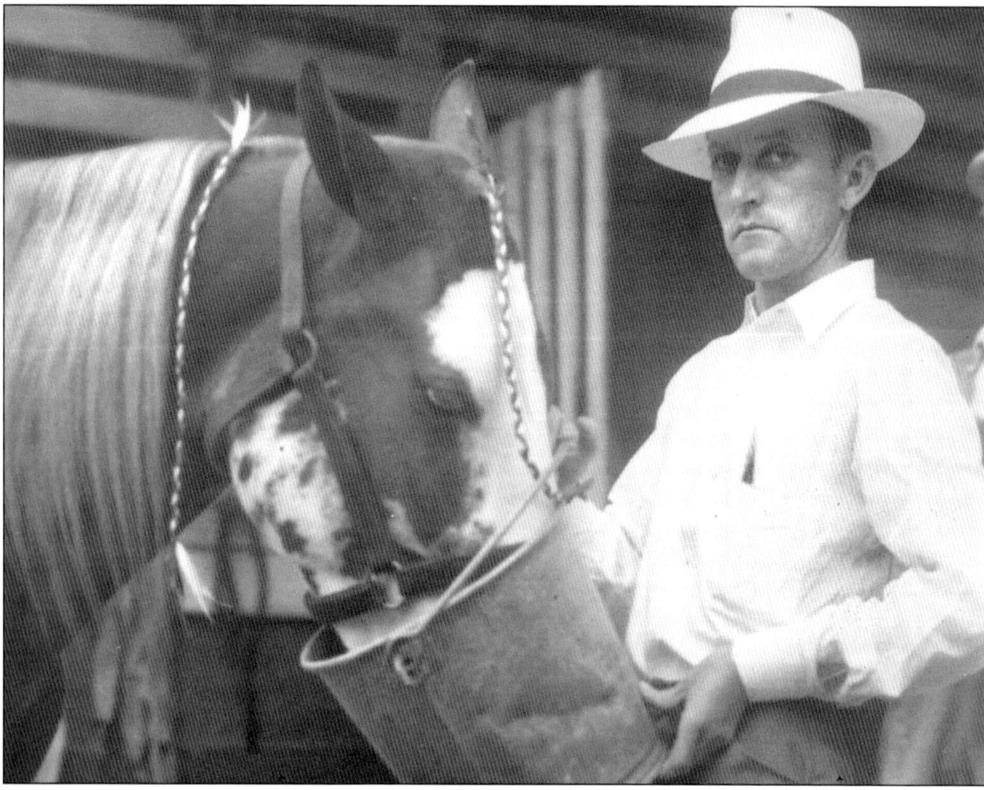

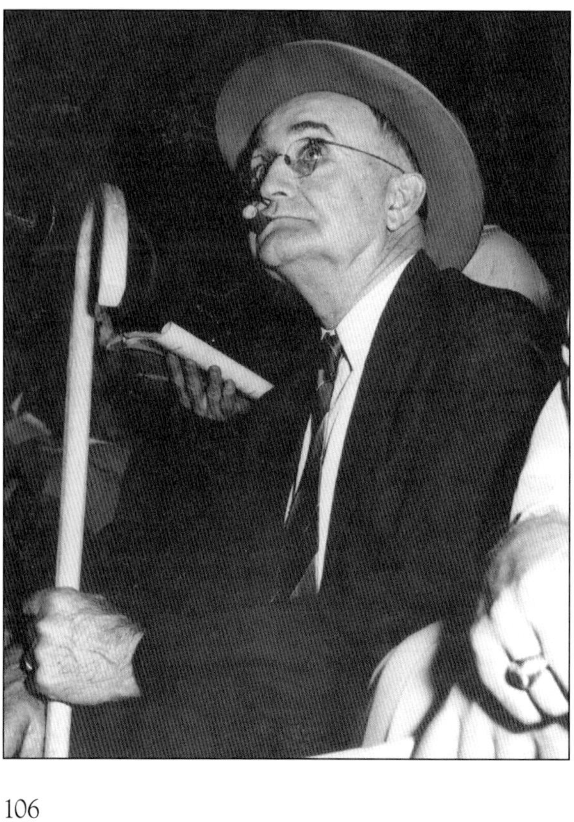

Tennessee Walking Horse trainer Steve Hill holds a bucket for the mare Destiny at his farm in Coffee County. Hill emerged as one of the top trainers during the 1940s and 1950s. He won his first Grand Championship with Midnight Merry in 1949. He also won a record three consecutive times from 1951 to 1953 with Talk of the Town. (Courtesy of Gore Center.)

Jimmy Joe Murray of Lewisburg attends the Murray Walking Horse sale on July 15, 1945. Murray was well known in the Tennessee Walking Horse industry. A successful farmer, he joined auctioneer and show announcer Jim McCord and Gov. Henry Horton to lobby for the 1929 establishment of a federal dairy demonstration facility in Marshall County. (Courtesy of Gore Center.)

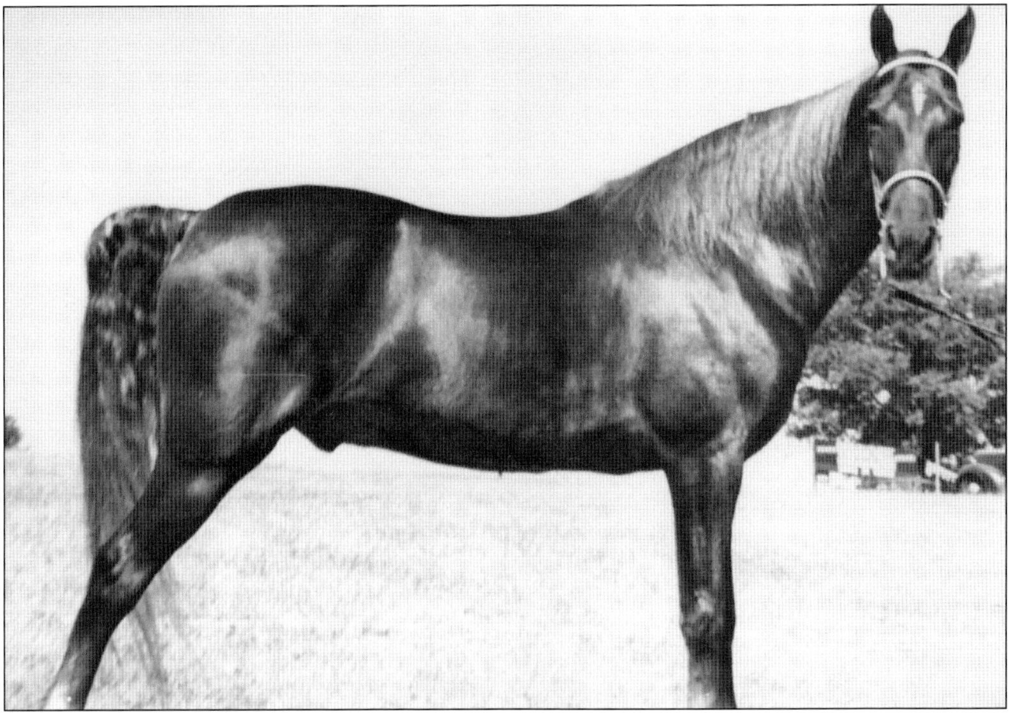

The Tennessee Walking Horse gelding G-Man, one of Wilson's Allen's many offspring, was one of several horses who helped build the popularity of the breed in the post–World War II era. Tennessee Walkers are encouraged to stand camped out, with their hind legs stretched out behind the perpendicular. (Courtesy of Gore Center.)

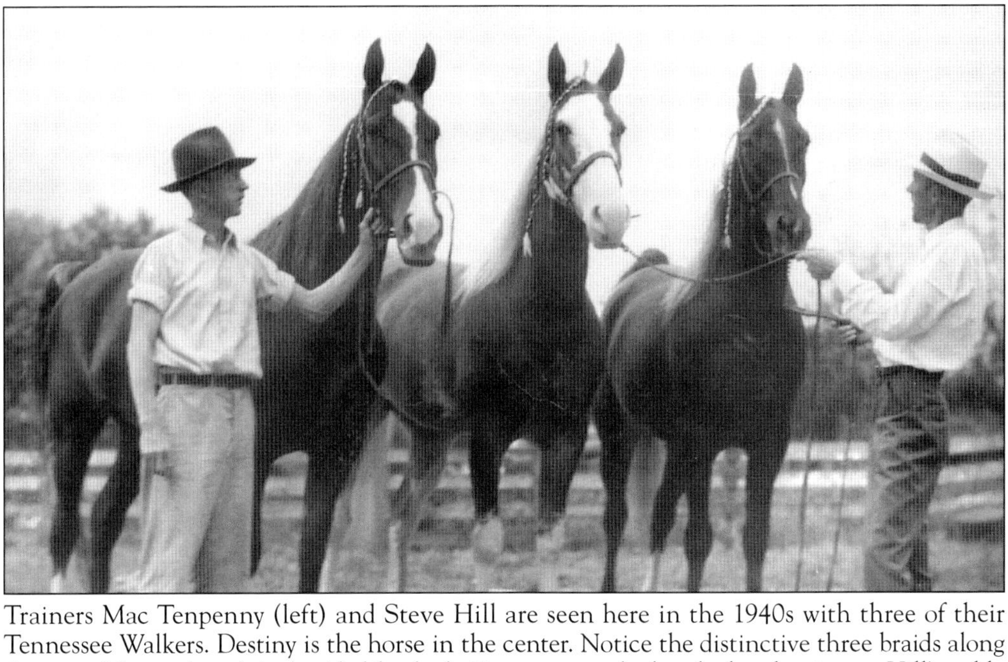

Trainers Mac Tenpenny (left) and Steve Hill are seen here in the 1940s with three of their Tennessee Walkers. Destiny is the horse in the center. Notice the distinctive three braids along the top of the neck and the braided forelock. Tenpenny worked as the head trainer at Hill's stable in Coffee County. (Courtesy of Gore Center.)

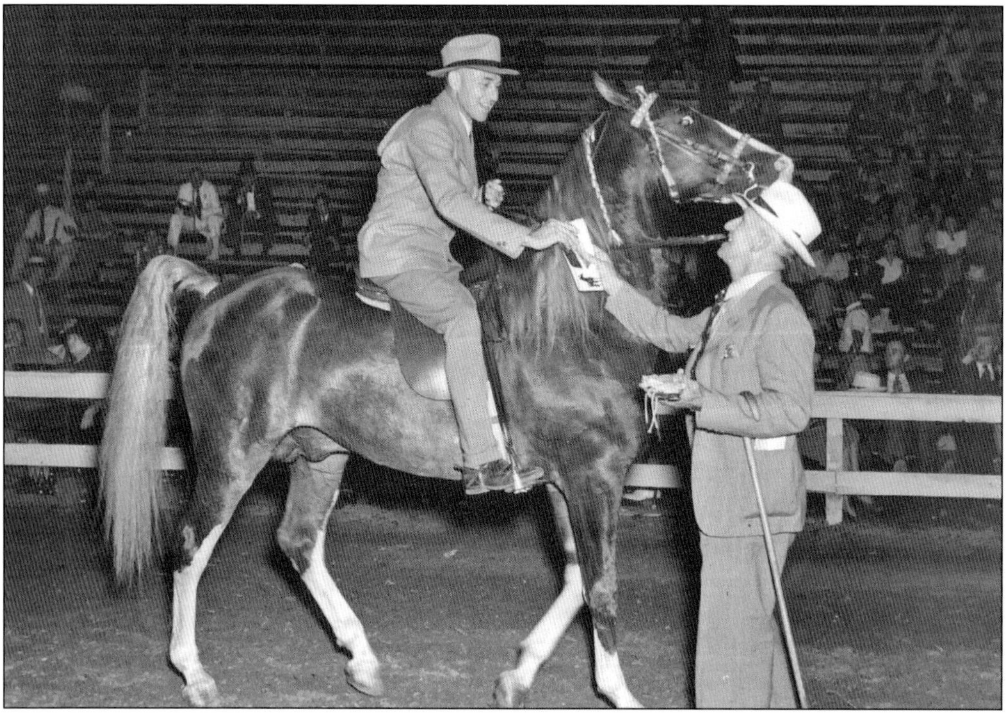

The winner of class 24 takes his ribbon from the ring master at this Tennessee Walking Horse National Celebration in the 1950s or 1960s. First-place winners often received a check in addition to a ribbon—or, even more special, a trophy. (Courtesy of Gore Center.)

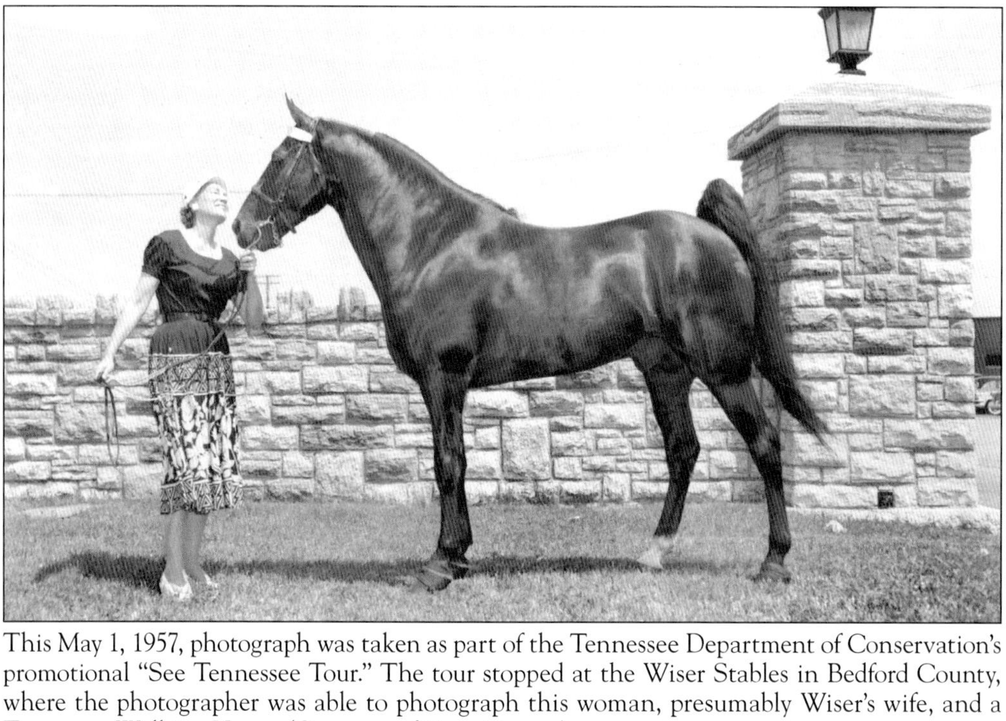

This May 1, 1957, photograph was taken as part of the Tennessee Department of Conservation's promotional "See Tennessee Tour." The tour stopped at the Wiser Stables in Bedford County, where the photographer was able to photograph this woman, presumably Wiser's wife, and a Tennessee Walking Horse. (Courtesy of Gore Center.)

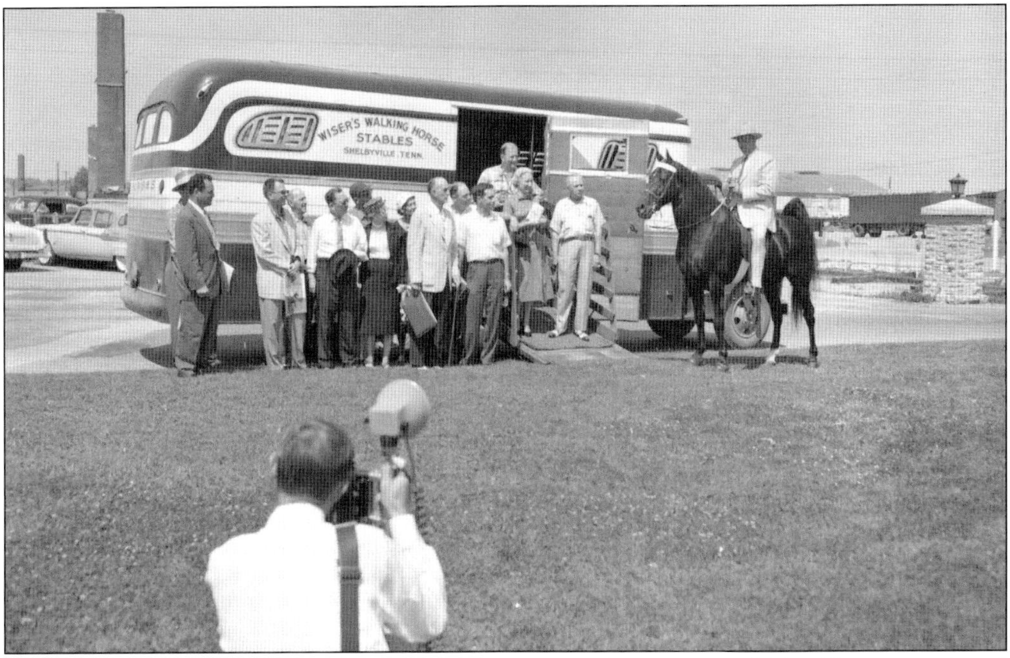

As part of the Tennessee Department of Conservation's promotional "See Tennessee Tour," the photographer not only took pictures of the horses but was also sometimes included in the photographs. This image is an excellent reminder of the large number of individuals who have worked in Middle Tennessee training barns over the last half-century. (Courtesy of TSLA.)

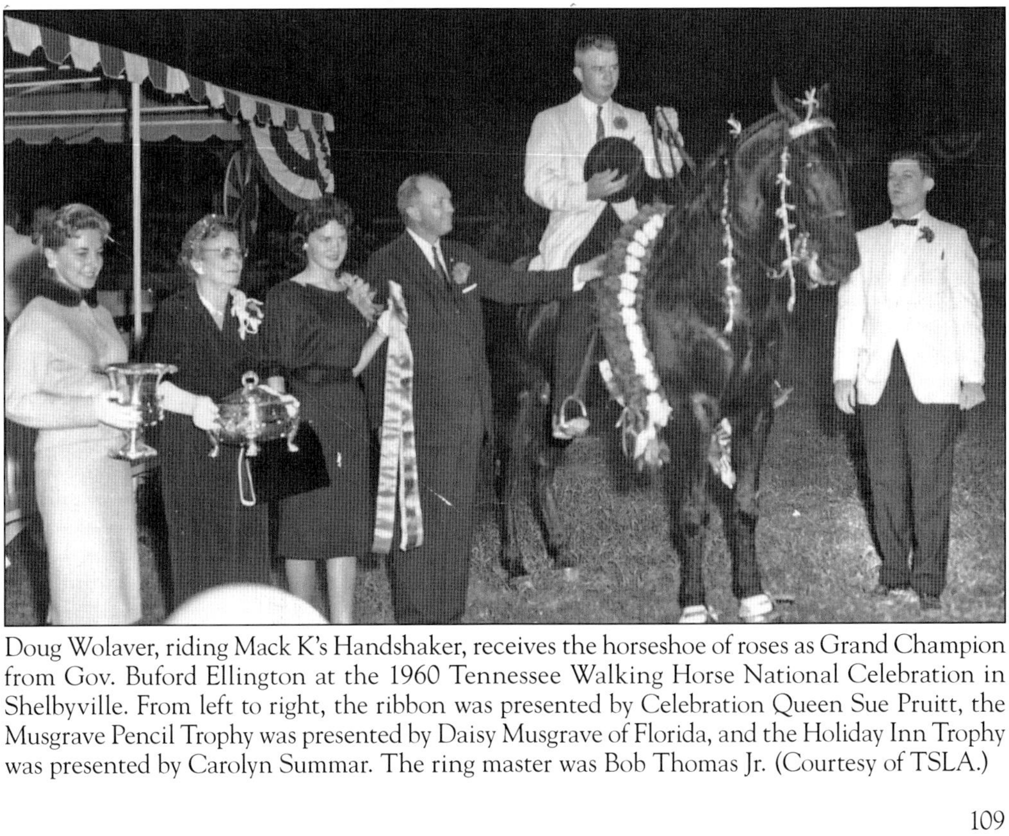

Doug Wolaver, riding Mack K's Handshaker, receives the horseshoe of roses as Grand Champion from Gov. Buford Ellington at the 1960 Tennessee Walking Horse National Celebration in Shelbyville. From left to right, the ribbon was presented by Celebration Queen Sue Pruitt, the Musgrave Pencil Trophy was presented by Daisy Musgrave of Florida, and the Holiday Inn Trophy was presented by Carolyn Summar. The ring master was Bob Thomas Jr. (Courtesy of TSLA.)

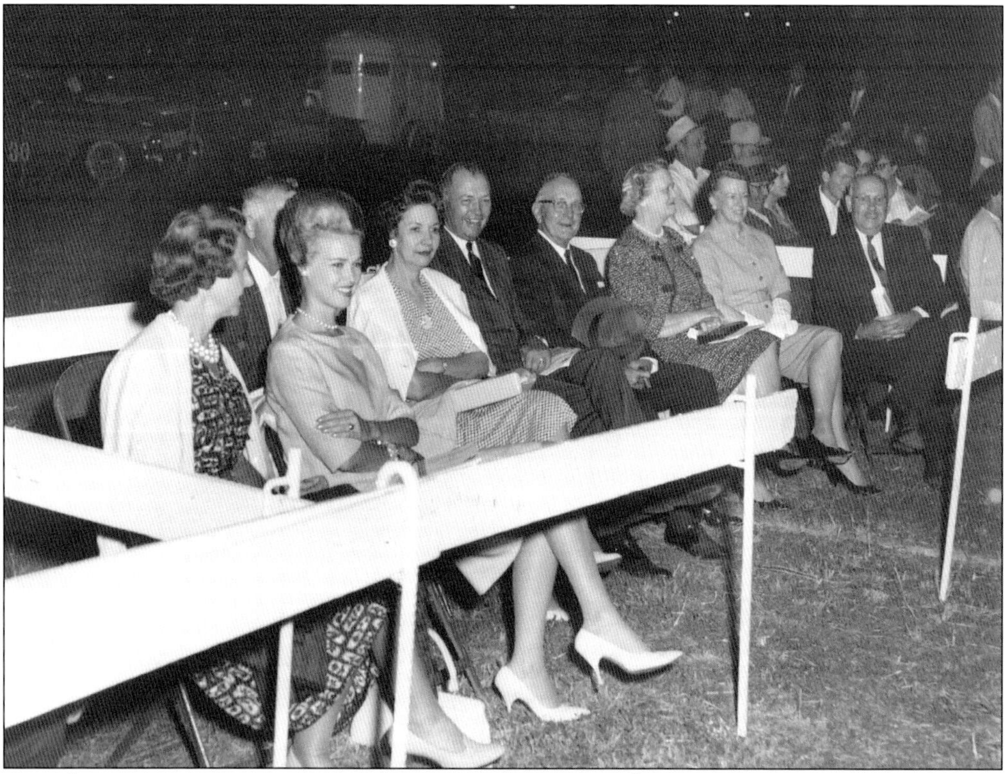

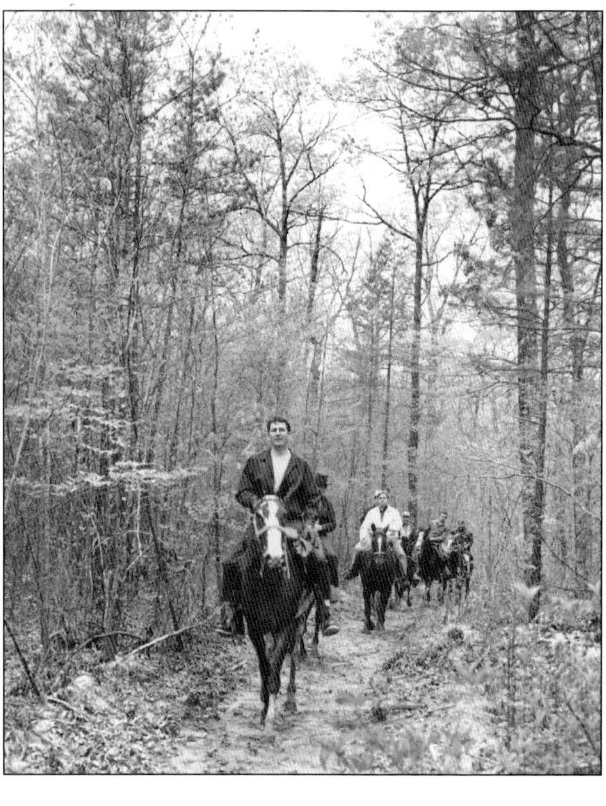

At a local Tennessee Walking Horse show in Lewisburg around 1960, the photographer found the show's guests at the center of the arena. Pictured from left to right are unidentified, Ann Ellington, Gov. Buford Ellington (who served from 1959 to 1963 and from 1967 to 1971), Mrs. Buford Ellington, and Conservation Commissioner J. Brents McBride. (Courtesy of TSLA.)

Gov. Winfield Dunn (who served from 1971 to 1975) shows that support for the Tennessee Walking Horse could cross party lines. Dunn was a Walking Horse owner. Like previous Middle Tennessee politicians, he tried to meet as many constituents as possible, and large-group horseback rides provided ample opportunity for mingling. (Courtesy of TSLA.)

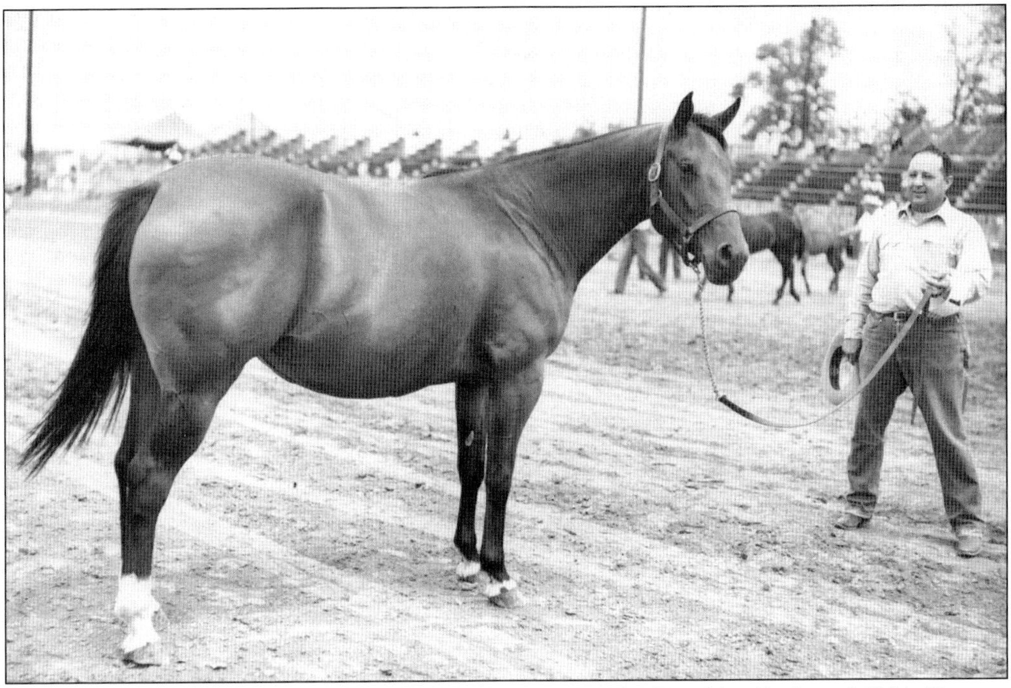

This horse was the Grand Champion Quarter Horse at the Franklin Rodeo of 1954. Quarter Horses are known for their muscular shoulders and hindquarters, as can be seen in this image, which allow them to better secure the roped steer or cow for the cowboy. (Courtesy of TSLA.)

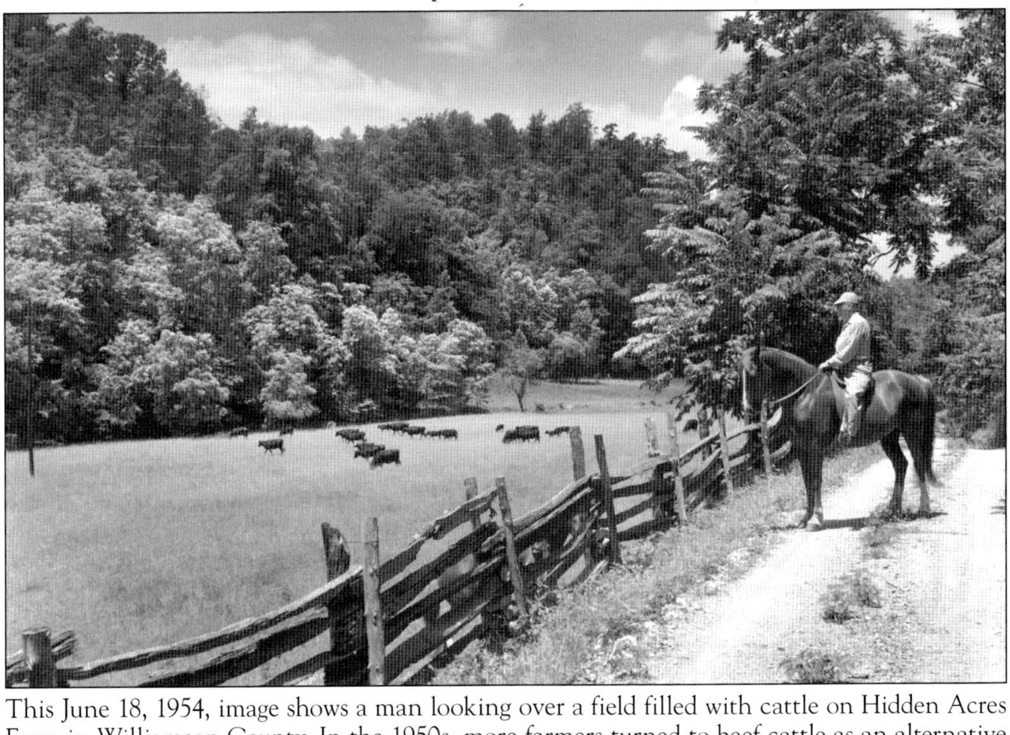

This June 18, 1954, image shows a man looking over a field filled with cattle on Hidden Acres Farm in Williamson County. In the 1950s, more farmers turned to beef cattle as an alternative to other livestock, thus increasing the need for good cow horses. (Courtesy of TSLA.)

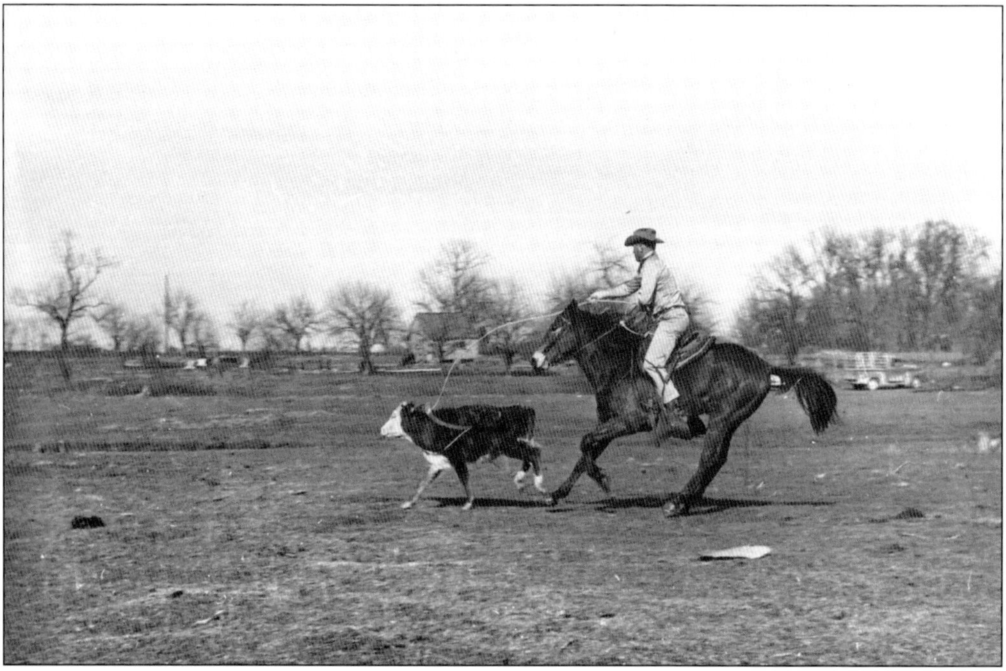

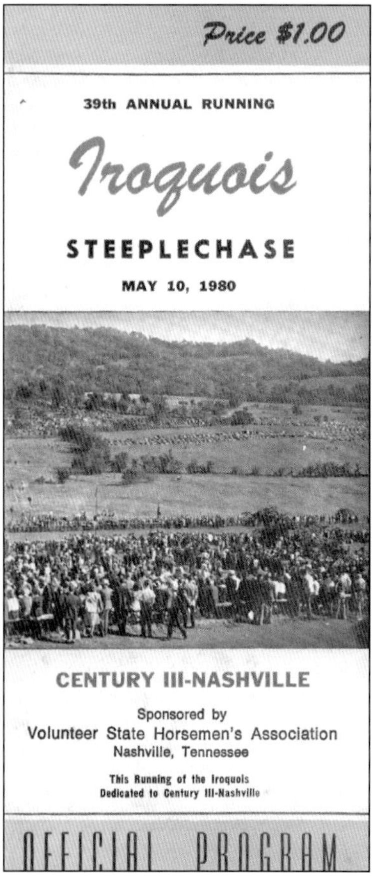

The unidentified man in this February 23, 1949, photograph is roping a calf on horseback at the John Fowlkes Ranch in Franklin. This photograph clearly shows the speed, agility, and strength required of Quarter Horses. (Courtesy of TSLA.)

This 1952 program from the Iroquois Steeplechase signals the beginning of a new era for Thoroughbreds in Middle Tennessee. Although anti-gambling laws still effectively outlawed flat racing, the region's premier steeplechase became nationally known thanks to Calvin Houghland, George Sloan, and Guilford Dudley, who rode their Nashville horses at other races around the country. (Courtesy of Gore Center.)

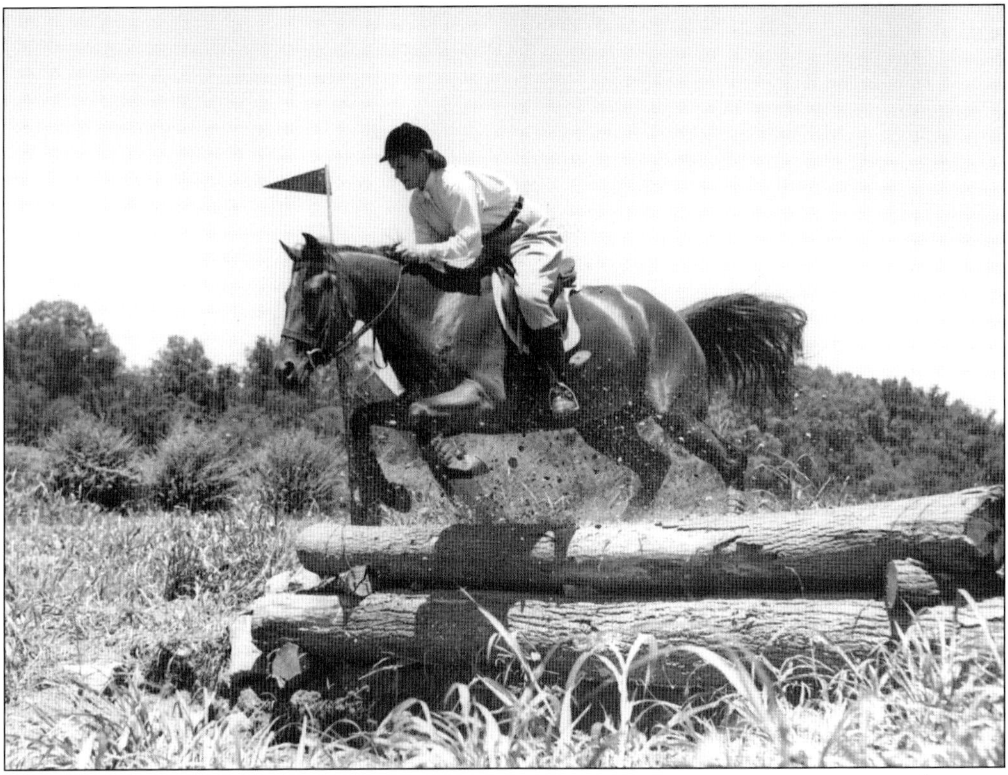

The 1953 "Horse Sense" Tournament was a one-day eventing type trial. The competitors, such as Kernan Regen, pictured here on Stutibev, had to be prepared to gallop and jump across varied terrain, and their horses had to perform a precise pattern of dressage movements and negotiate a show-jumping course. (Courtesy of Gore Center.)

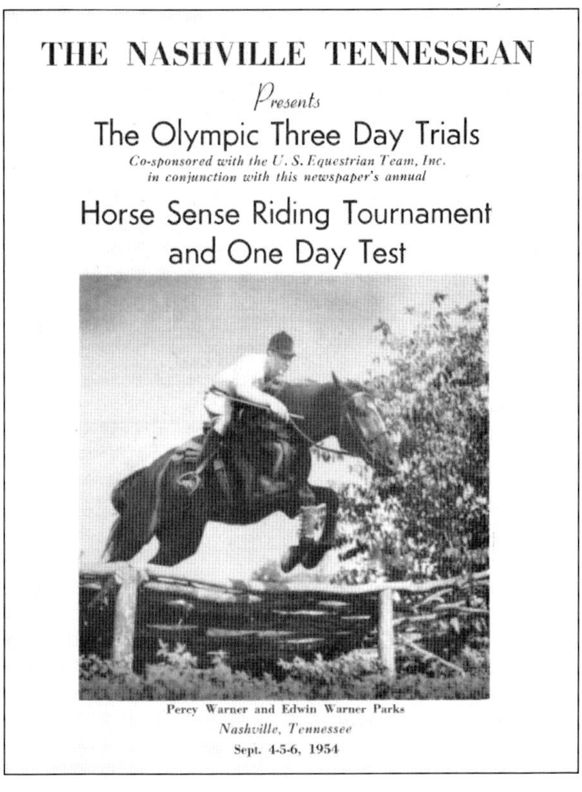

THE NASHVILLE TENNESSEAN

Presents

The Olympic Three Day Trials

Co-sponsored with the U. S. Equestrian Team, Inc.
in conjunction with this newspaper's annual

Horse Sense Riding Tournament
and One Day Test

Percy Warner and Edwin Warner Parks
Nashville, Tennessee
Sept. 4-5-6, 1954

This program from the 1954 Olympic three-day trial is a nationally significant piece of history. At this event, Middle Tennesseans had the opportunity to pit their horses against the best horses produced by the military's system. The event also included several female riders. The only downside of the weekend was the unseasonably high temperatures, which caused several horses to collapse and die from heat exhaustion. (Courtesy of Gore Center.)

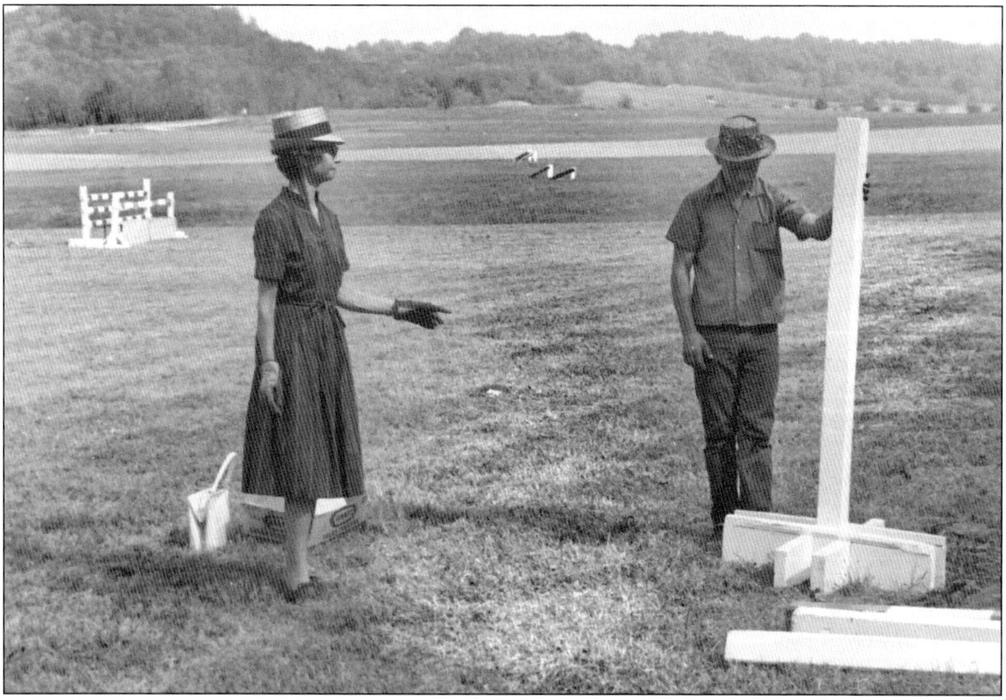

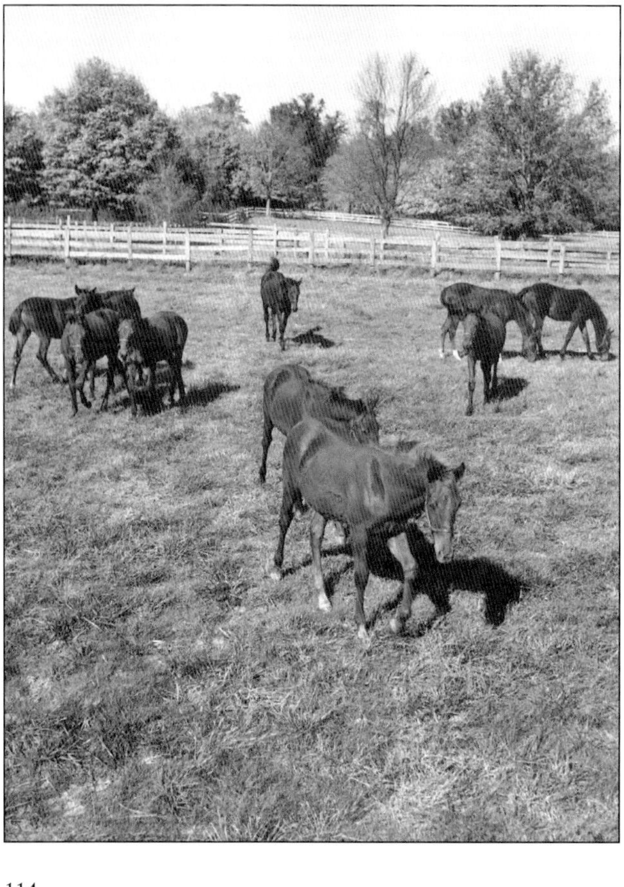

In this August 1954 photograph, Margaret Lindsley Warden directs the setting of the stadium course at the three-day trial. Course designs have become increasingly sophisticated during the last 25 years. The Franklin-based company Jumps by Fuzzy, owned by Fuzzy Mayo, is one of the nation's largest jump-building and course-designing companies for hunter and jumper competitions. Mayo rode in the Interschool Riding Tournaments as a child. (Courtesy of Gore Center.)

These Thoroughbred weanlings at Laura Branham's Foxland Hall represent the resurgence of racehorse breeding in Middle Tennessee. The Branhams moved to Gallatin in the late 1920s and were part of the failed Grasslands venture at Fairview. The Foxland Hall Thoroughbred breeding program was successful. (Courtesy of TSLA.)

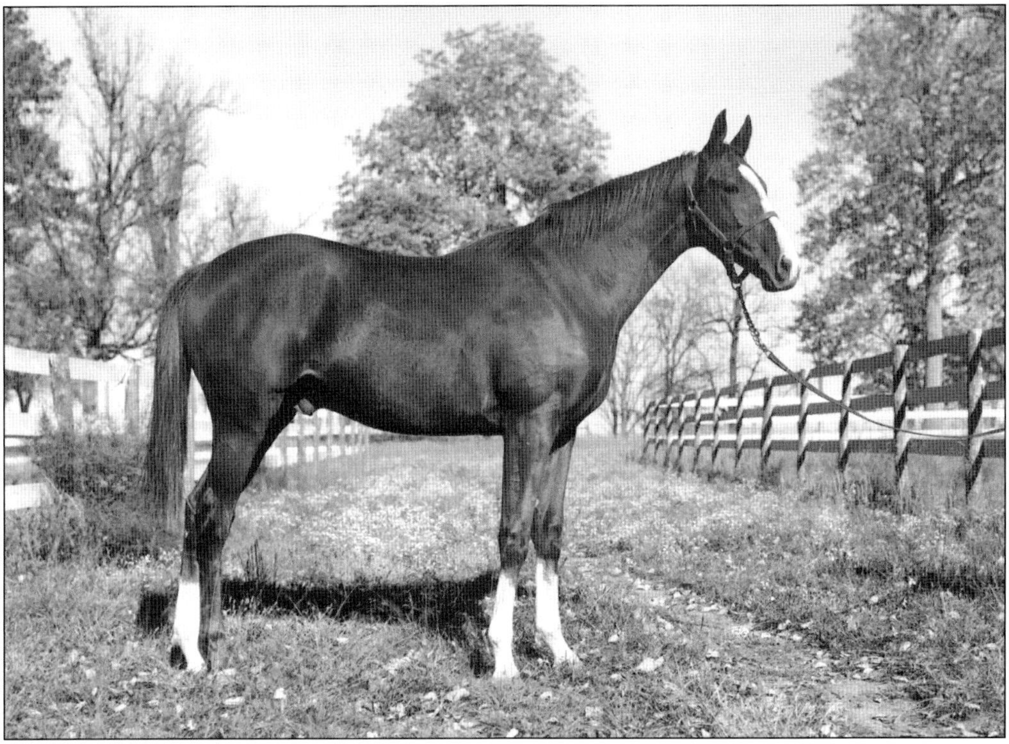

This Thoroughbred stallion, Joe's Choice, out of (mothered by) Ionia, (fathered) by Isolater, was owned by I. C. McMahan. In 1913, the McMahan family bought the historic Kennesaw Stud, built in 1856 outside Gallatin. They used it as a Thoroughbred breeding and training farm until it was sold in 2004 for residential and business development. (Courtesy of TSLA.)

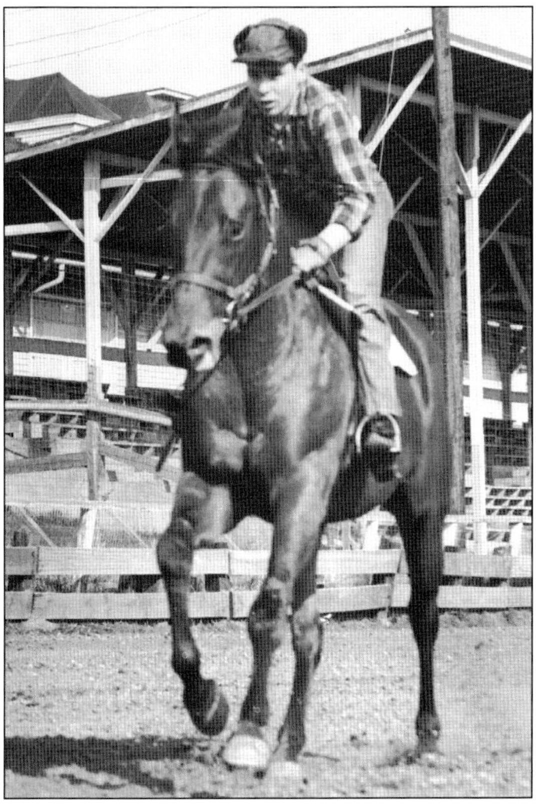

Johnny Pruitt, an exercise boy turning jockey, rides under the tutelage of trainer George C. White of Nashville in this February 1956 photograph. Although riding racehorses is a dangerous profession, many lightweight and courageous Middle Tennessee youths have begun careers as exercise riders, a tradition that dates to before the Civil War. (Courtesy of Gore Center.)

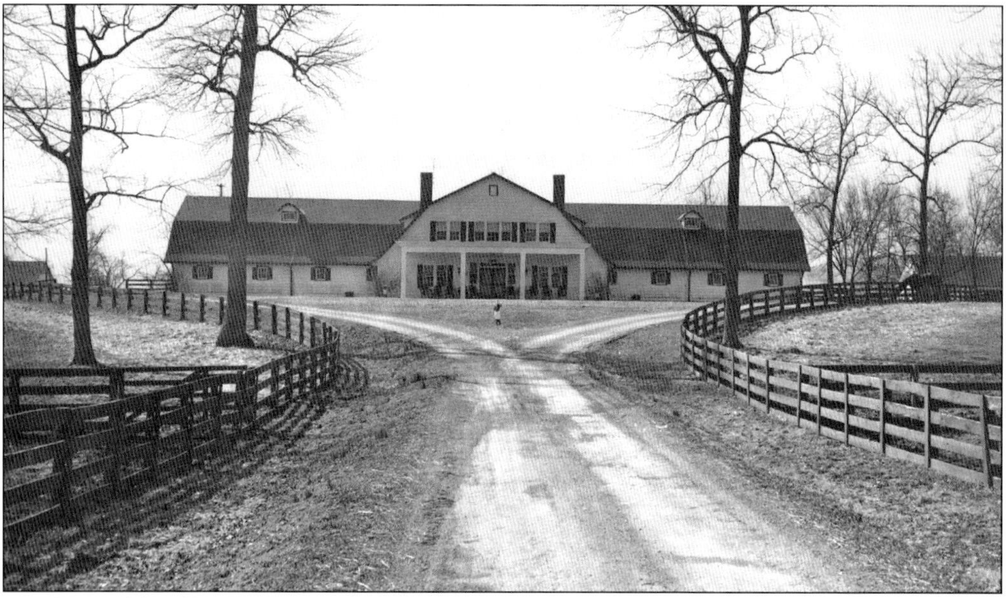

As Thoroughbred breeding rebounded in Middle Tennessee, older stables, such as the Saddlebred stud Maryland Farm, were converted into horse racing tracks. This 1960s photograph shows the main stable after its conversion into a Thoroughbred center by the Volunteer State Horseman's Association. The stable had also served as a Hereford cattle barn for five years before the conversion. (Courtesy of TSLA.)

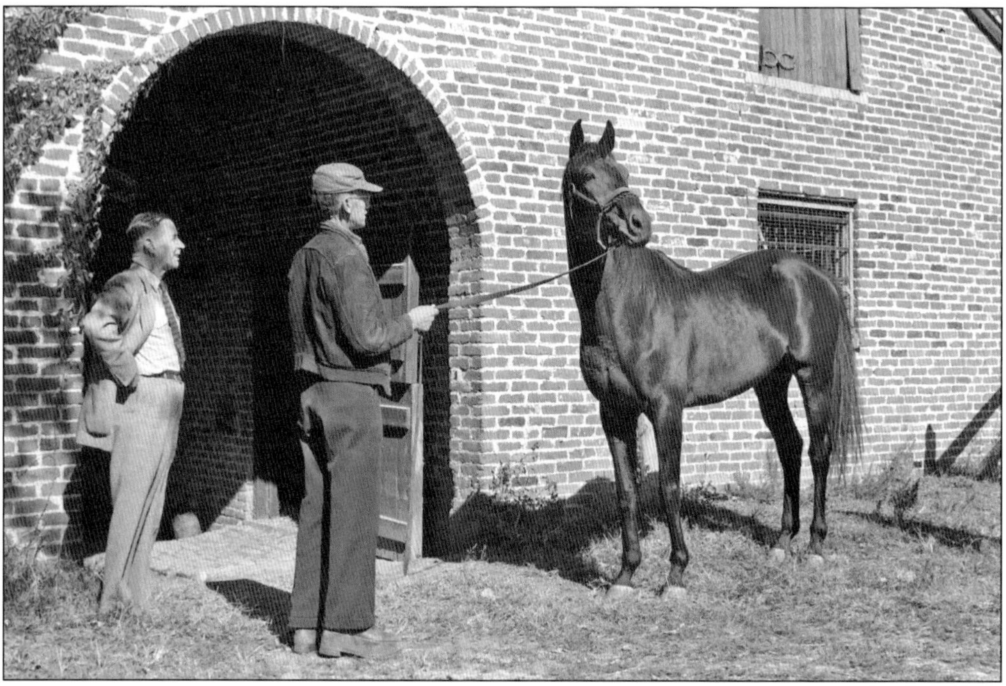

Another influential postwar Thoroughbred breeder was Col. Campbell Brown (left), president of the Tennessee Thoroughbred Club. His farm manager, Clay Stone (right), is with the stallion Shadows Start (fathered) by Hoop Jr., out of (mothered by) Night Shadow, (fathered) by Man O'Night. (Courtesy of TSLA.)

This photograph was taken during the 1960s at Cothran Campbell's Shoe String Farm in Franklin. Campbell's father owned several prizewinning saddle horses, including Satin Star. In the early 1940s, Campbell established Dogwood Stable in Aiken, South Carolina, where James B. Tafel, the owner and breeder of the 2007 Kentucky Derby winner Street Sense, was first introduced to racing. (Courtesy of Gore Center.)

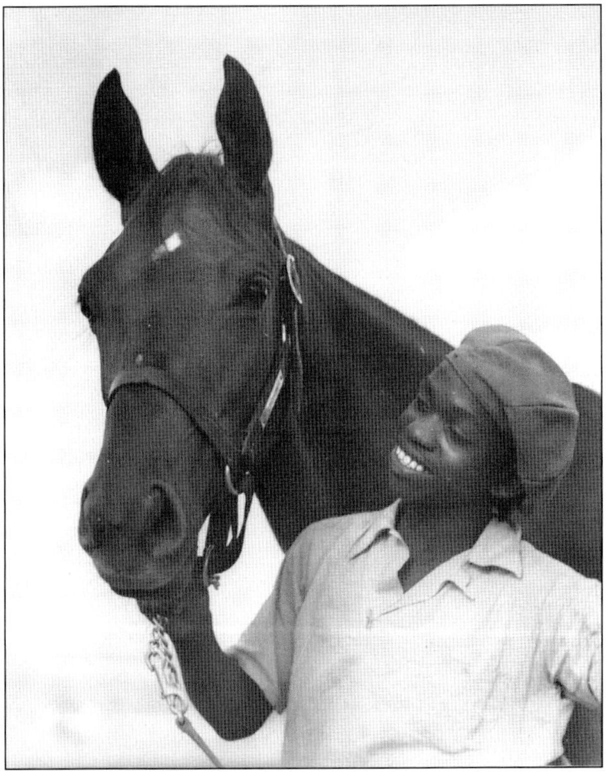

In Brentwood, Calvin Houghland's 1940s Thoroughbred weanlings enjoyed standing for the camera at his Bright Hour Farm. The property was named for the horse he rode to victory in the Tennessee Timber Toppers steeplechase at Overton Downs in 1932. (Courtesy of TSLA.)

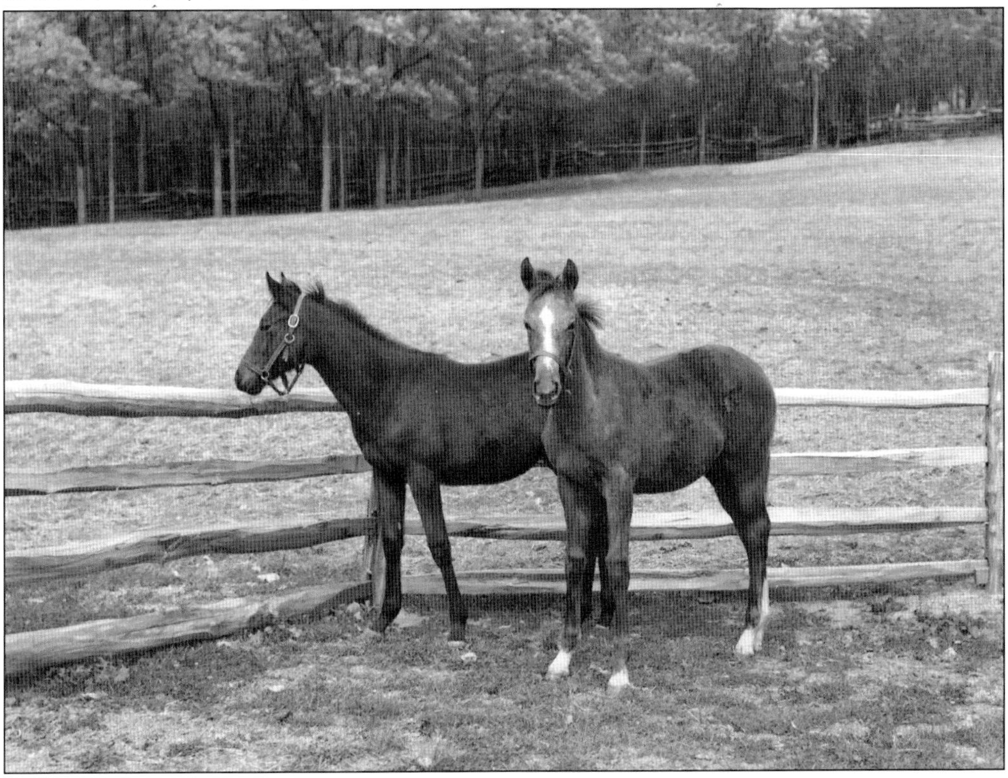

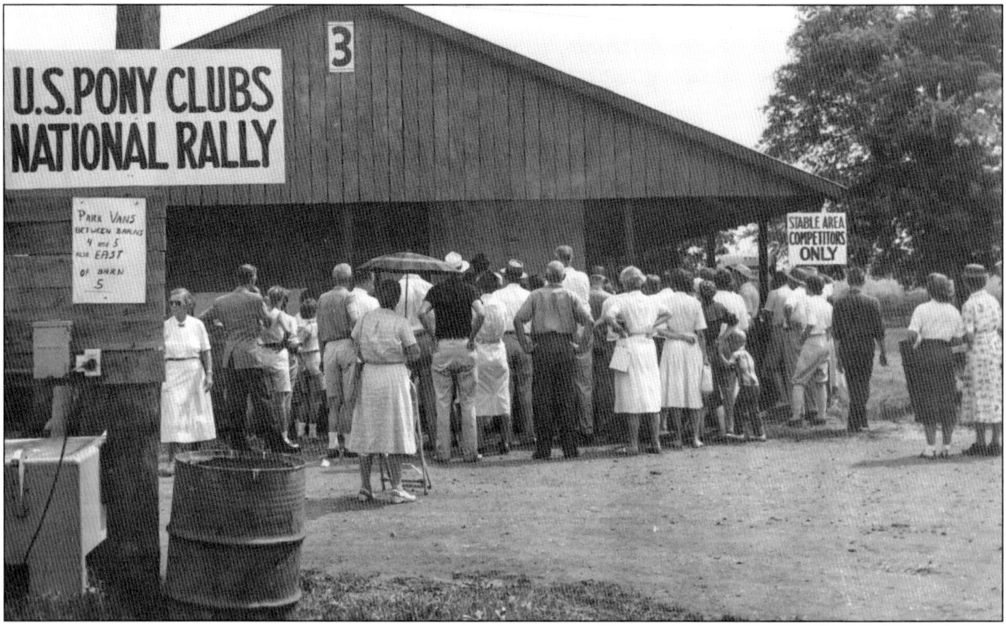

The final scores are posted at the stables during the U.S. Pony Clubs' national rally in July 1959. The rally was hosted by the Middle Tennessee Pony Club and was held at Maryland Farms and Percy Warner Park in Brentwood. Pony clubbers have to qualify for the championships each year, and they can have no parental help in caring for or riding their mounts while they are competing. (Courtesy of Gore Center.)

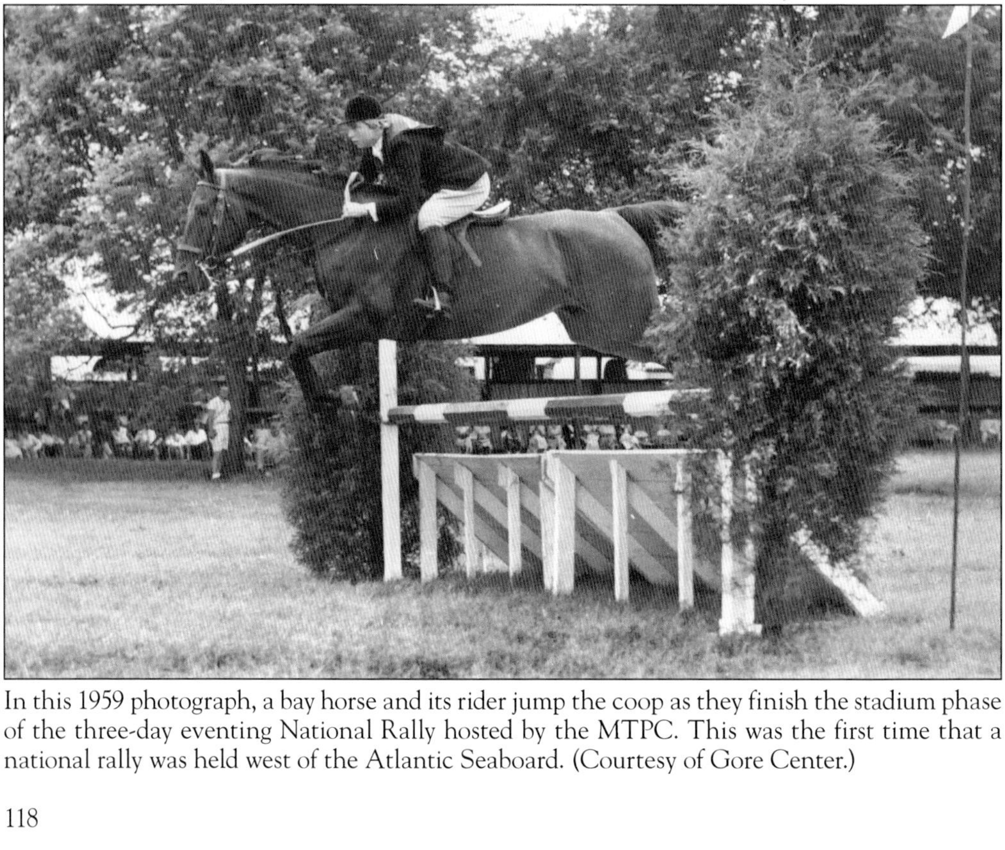
In this 1959 photograph, a bay horse and its rider jump the coop as they finish the stadium phase of the three-day eventing National Rally hosted by the MTPC. This was the first time that a national rally was held west of the Atlantic Seaboard. (Courtesy of Gore Center.)

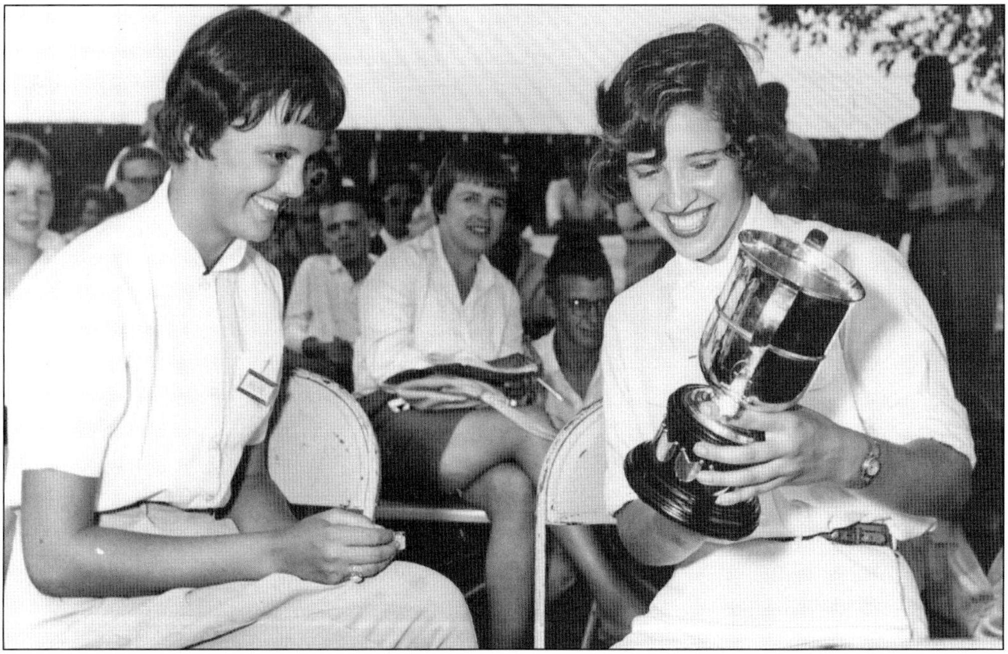

Above, A-level Florence Newbern of West Tennessee Pony Club looks on as Joy Yearwood of MTPC admires her trophy at the 1959 National Rally in Brentwood. The pony club used a series of levels—D, C, B, and A—to chart a child's progression in riding and knowledge. Below, Nashville's Bold Minstrel and his owner, William D. Haggard III, begin their journey to a 1959 Pan American Games team silver in eventing. In 1963, they took home a team gold. Haggard allowed eventer Mike Plumb to ride Bold Minstrel to a team gold in the 1964 Olympics, and show jumper William Steinkraus rode the horse to a team silver at the 1967 Pan American Games. Bold Minstrel is the only American horse to have competed in two different world-class equestrian events. (Courtesy of Gore Center.)

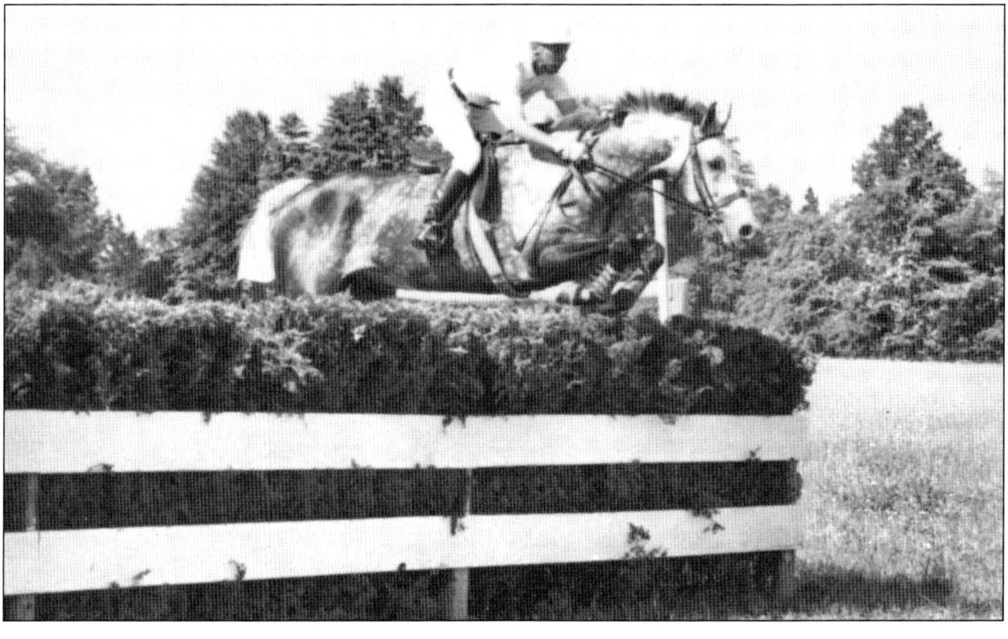

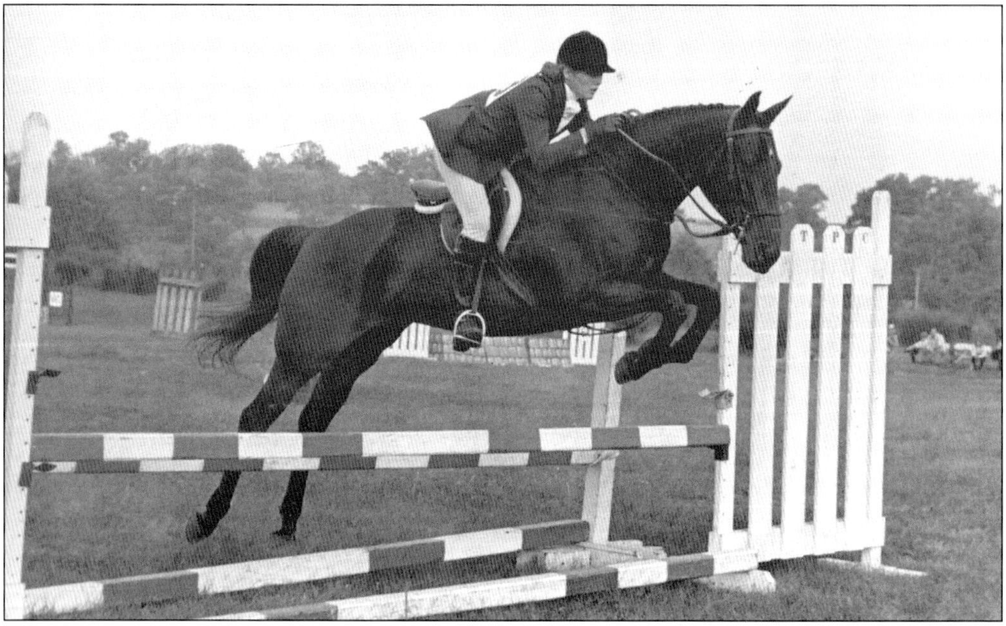

This 1964 photograph of Charlene McMurray on Traveler in the show jumping phase of the *Tennessean* Horse Sense one-day trial shows the growth of the event. Organizers condensed what was normally a three-day event into one day to speed up the competition and make it less difficult for the horses and riders. (Courtesy of Gore Center; photograph by Harriet Benton.)

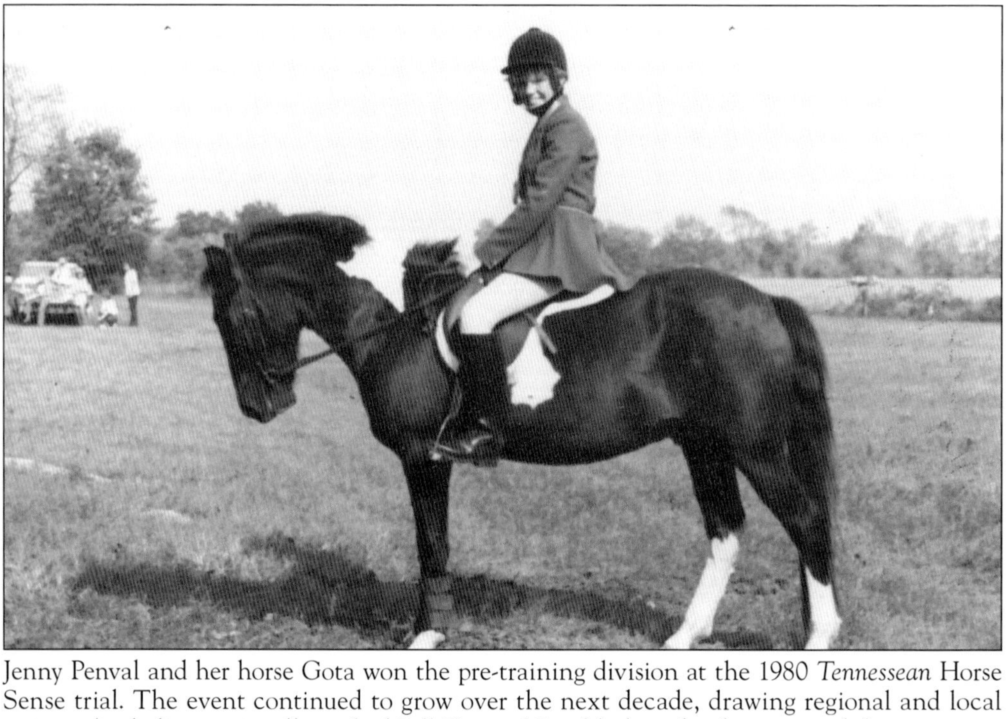

Jenny Penval and her horse Gota won the pre-training division at the 1980 *Tennessean* Horse Sense trial. The event continued to grow over the next decade, drawing regional and local trainers (including nationally ranked Bill Hoos of Franklin) to the dressage and show jumping phases at Brownland Farm in Franklin and to the cross-country course at Percy Warner Park. (Courtesy of Gore Center.)

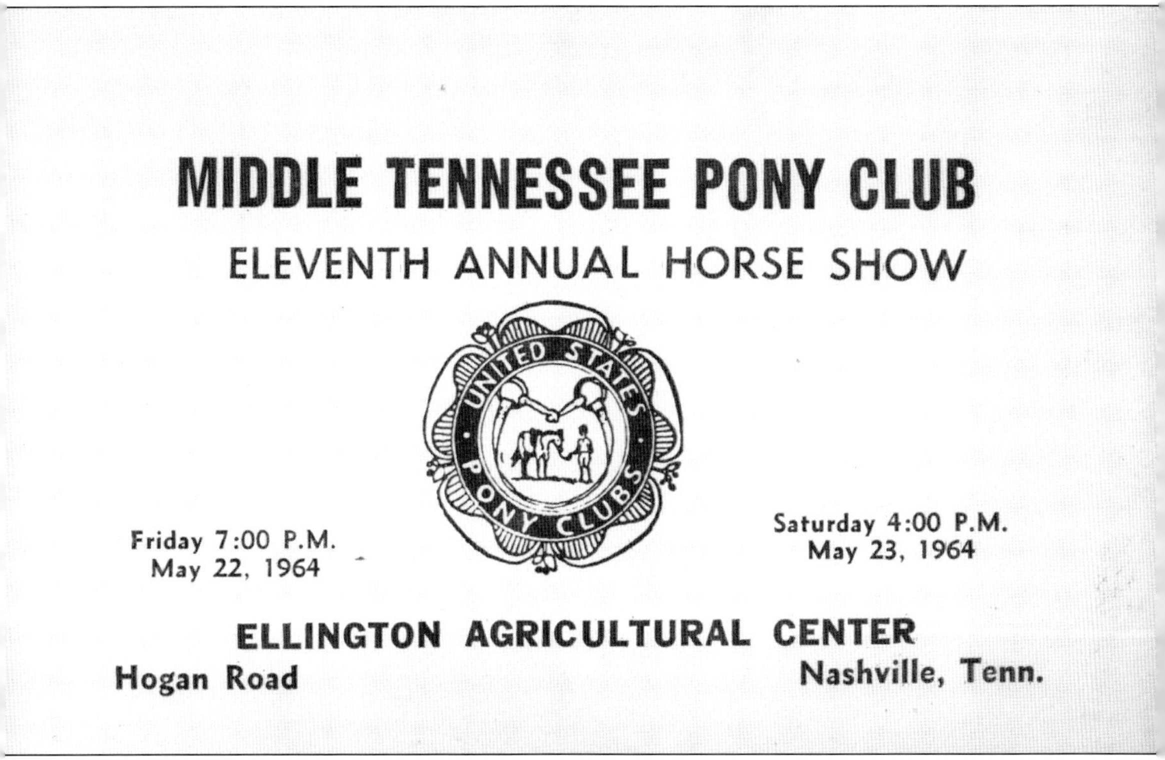
MIDDLE TENNESSEE PONY CLUB
ELEVENTH ANNUAL HORSE SHOW
UNITED STATES PONY CLUBS
Friday 7:00 P.M.
May 22, 1964
Saturday 4:00 P.M.
May 23, 1964
ELLINGTON AGRICULTURAL CENTER
Hogan Road
Nashville, Tenn.

This 1964 advertising card from the Middle Tennessee Pony Club's horse show represents yet another facet of the club during the 1960s to 1970s, when it was under the direction of Margaret Lindsley Warden. Almost all of the horse show's classes, which ranged from costume classes to games and equitation, were open to the public. The shows raised money to help pay for members' expenses, such as the cost of attending the regional and national rallies. By 1964, Warden's dream of introducing Middle Tennessee to forward riding was coming true. At the same time, these horse shows introduced more people to jumping and began a period of extended growth for the pony club. It eventually split into several different clubs, but, under Warden's leadership, they remained united as branches of the larger Middle Tennessee Pony Club. Ellington Agricultural Center was a popular location for indoor or limited-space horse shows. (Courtesy of Gore Center.)

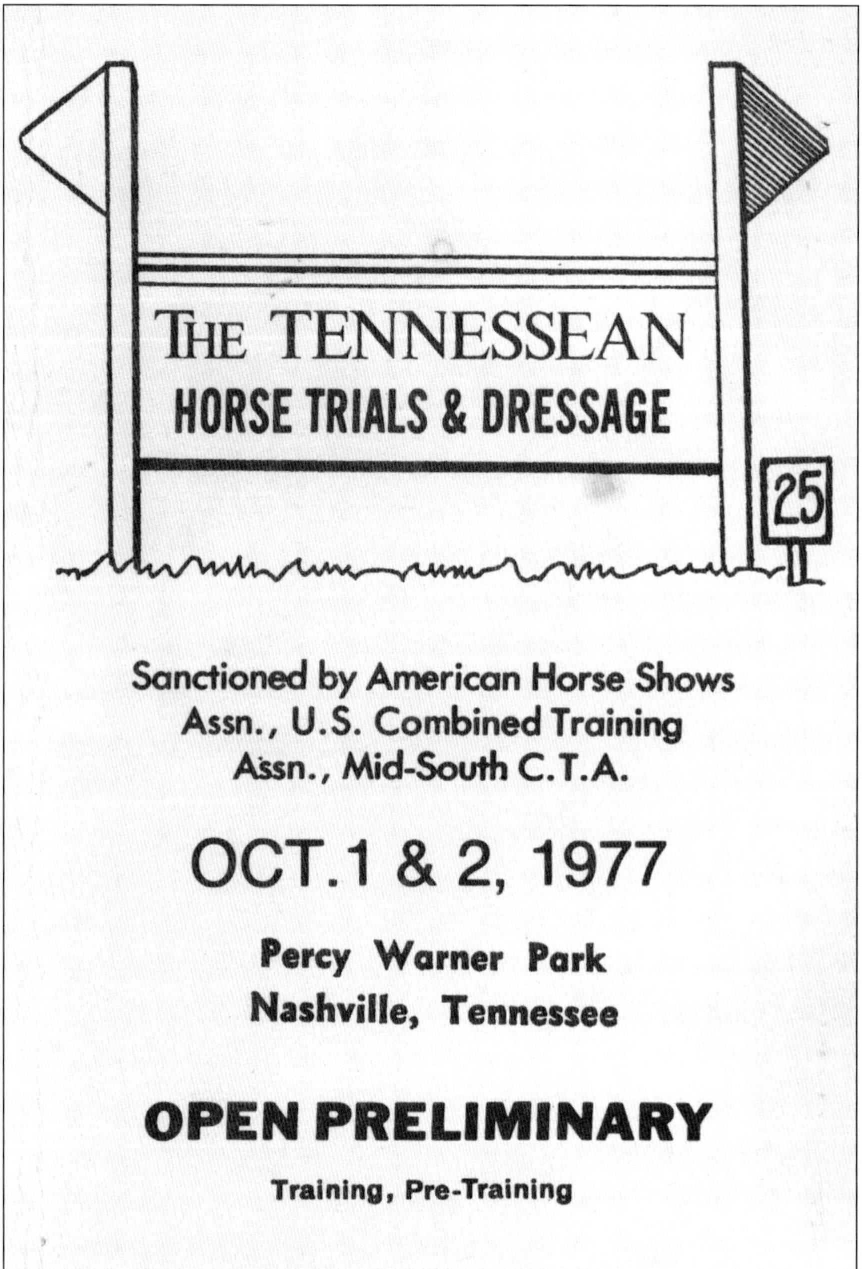

This 1977 show bill lists the *Tennessean* Dressage Trial, also begun by Margaret Lindsley Warden, which ran concurrently with the Horse Trial. Dressage riders follow a prescribed pattern of circles, lines, half circles, and diagonals. The standard ring size is 60 meters by 40 meters, with letters spaced equidistantly along the edge to guide the riders. The judge sits along the short end in order to have the best view. Each rider's movements are judged on a scale of 1 to 10, as are the rider's position and the horse's overall gaits, impulsion, and submission. The marks are then totaled, and class winners are those with the highest scores. In contrast to Thoroughbred and Standardbred racing and gaited horse shows, any breed or size of horse can compete in dressage. (Courtesy of Gore Center.)

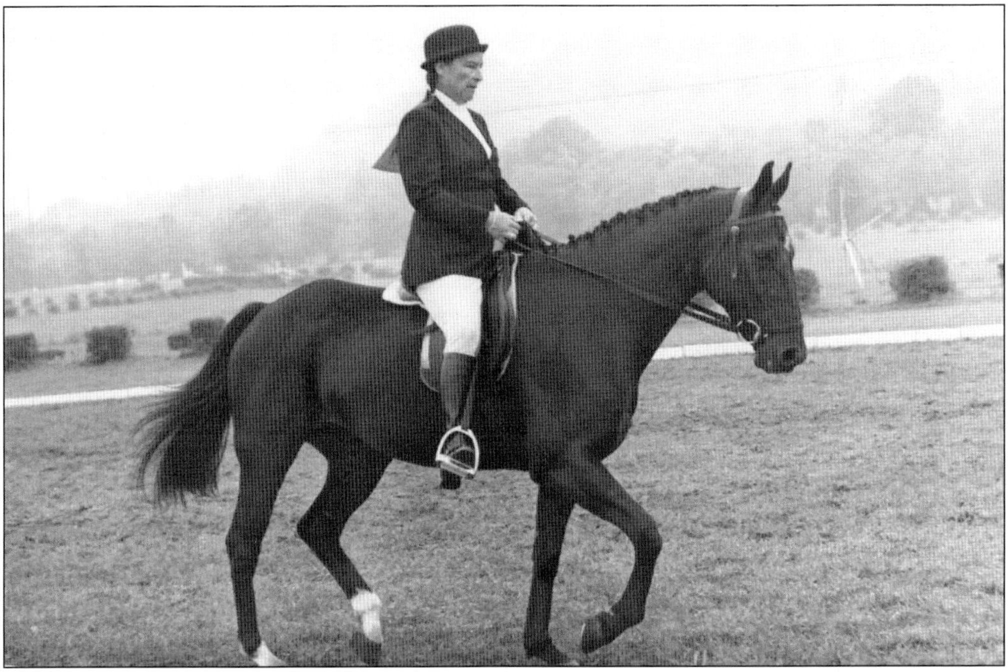

Susan Munro rides Boston Ann at the seventh annual *Tennessean* Dressage Show in 1973. The annual competition was held for many years at Percy Warner Park in Nashville. The hills that frame the steeplechase and eventing courses are clearly visible in the background. (Courtesy of Gore Center.)

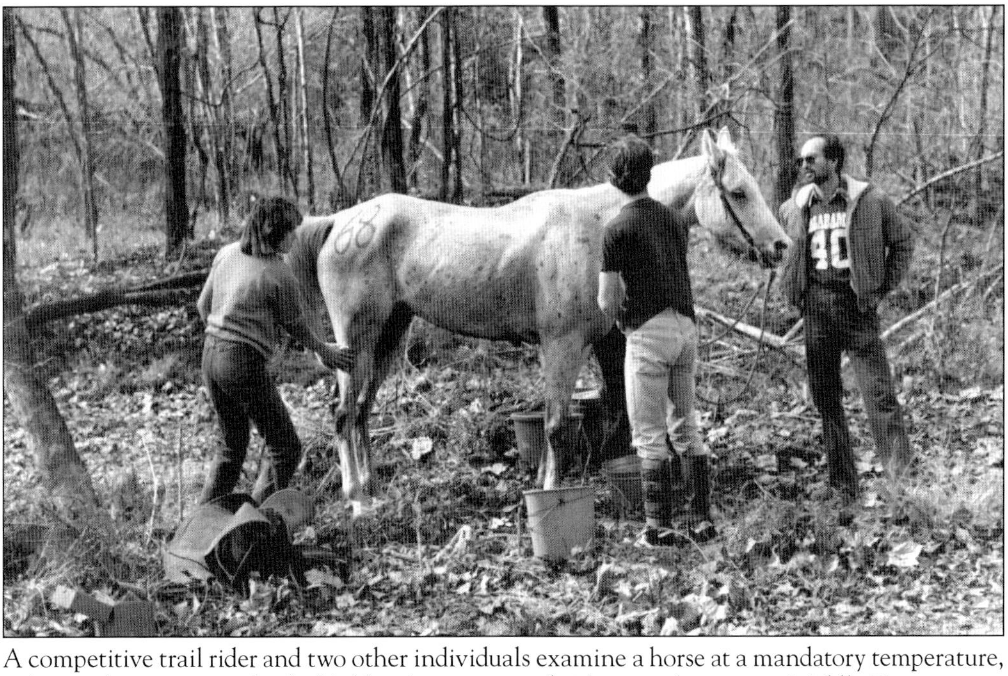

A competitive trail rider and two other individuals examine a horse at a mandatory temperature, pulse, and respiration check. Unlike the group trail rides popular among Middle Tennesseans in the first half of the century, these rides are judged against the clock and other competitors. (Courtesy of Gore Center.)

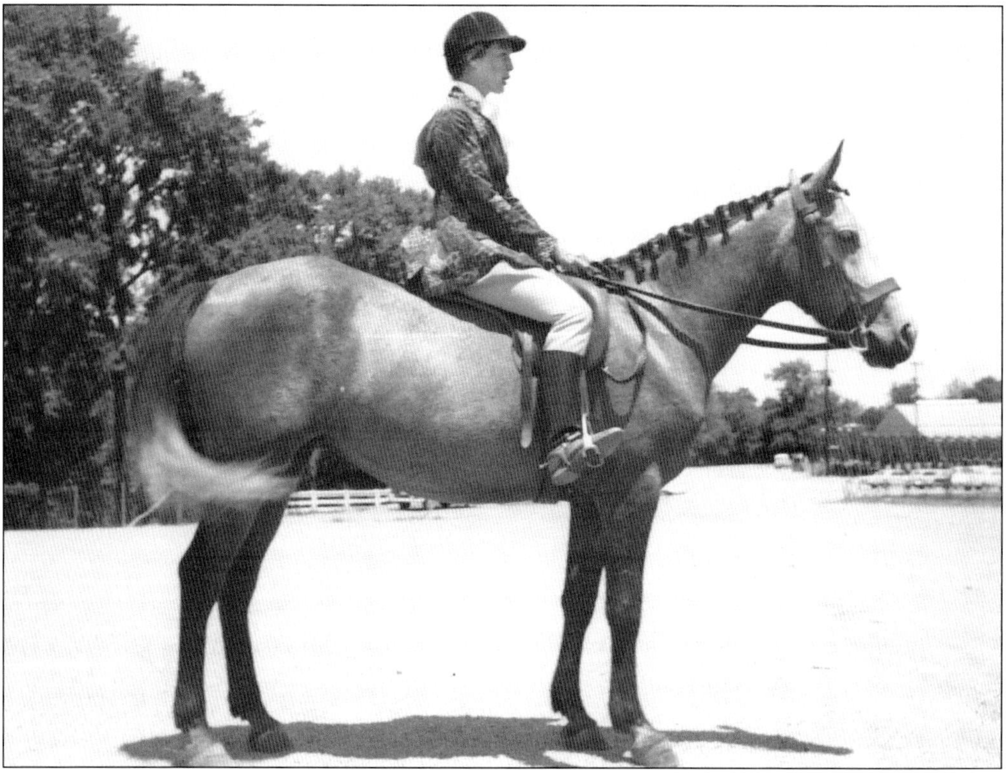

Armide, a three-year-old, hunter-type Arabian filly bred by Margaret Lindsley Warden, was ridden in the show ring by Polly Peach on July 21, 1962, at the West Meade show. Beginning the next year, with new owner Vicki Medlin, Armide won numerous hunter under saddle and hunter over fences awards at Middle Tennessee horse shows. (Courtesy of Gore Center.)

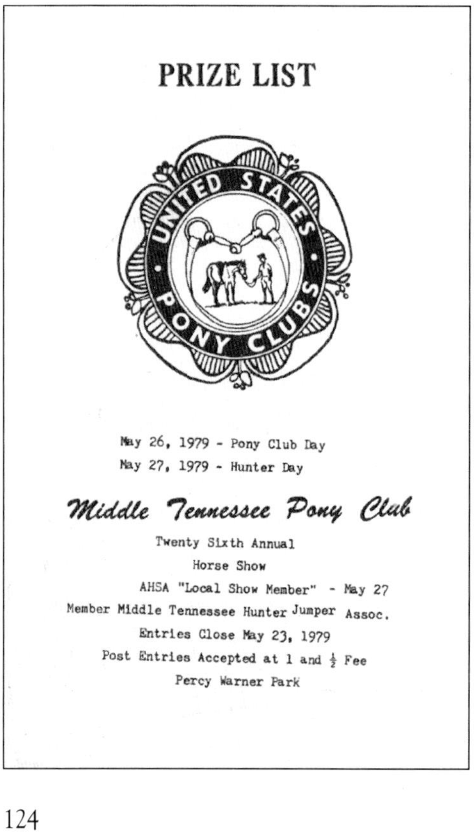

PRIZE LIST

UNITED STATES PONY CLUBS

May 26, 1979 - Pony Club Day
May 27, 1979 - Hunter Day

Middle Tennessee Pony Club

Twenty Sixth Annual
Horse Show
AHSA "Local Show Member" - May 27
Member Middle Tennessee Hunter Jumper Assoc.
Entries Close May 23, 1979
Post Entries Accepted at 1 and ½ Fee
Percy Warner Park

This 1979 show bill for the Middle Tennessee Pony Club's horse show demonstrates how much the hunter and jumper industry grew during the 1960s and 1970s. No longer was the horse show advertising a wide range of "fun" classes. The show had gained recognition from regional sport organizations, and its riders could earn points toward year-end awards. (Courtesy of Gore Center.)

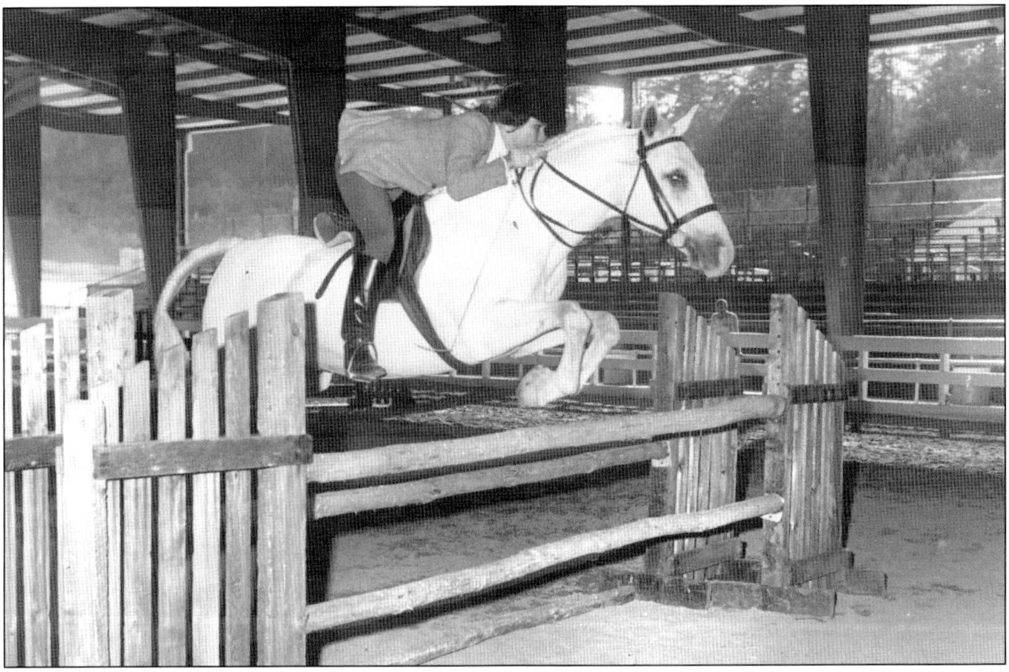

Tami Fleming jumps one of her mother's Travellers Rest Arabians, named Traveler, over a sizable oxer at their farm in Columbia. The family's connection to horse breeding dates to 1799 with the establishment of John Overton's Travellers Rest in Nashville. (Courtesy of Travellers Rest Plantation and Museum.)

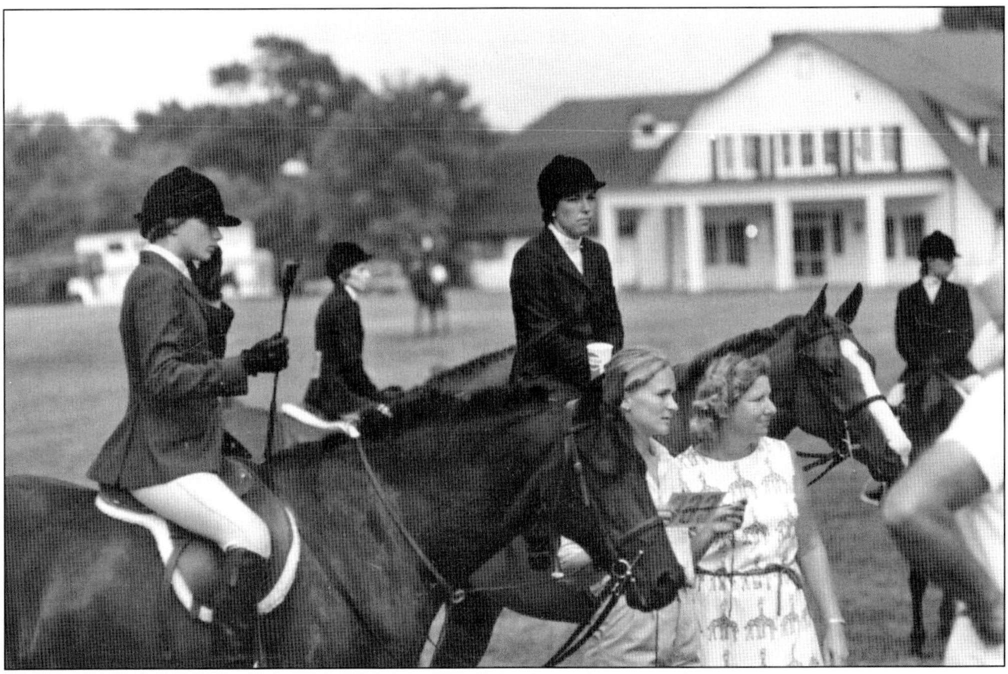

Two unidentified women, one of whom is most likely the trainer, stand among several mounted women at a Nashville area hunter show around 1980. Hunters are judged on style and jumpers are judged on speed. Most competitors at hunter and jumper shows are women. (Courtesy of Gore Center.)

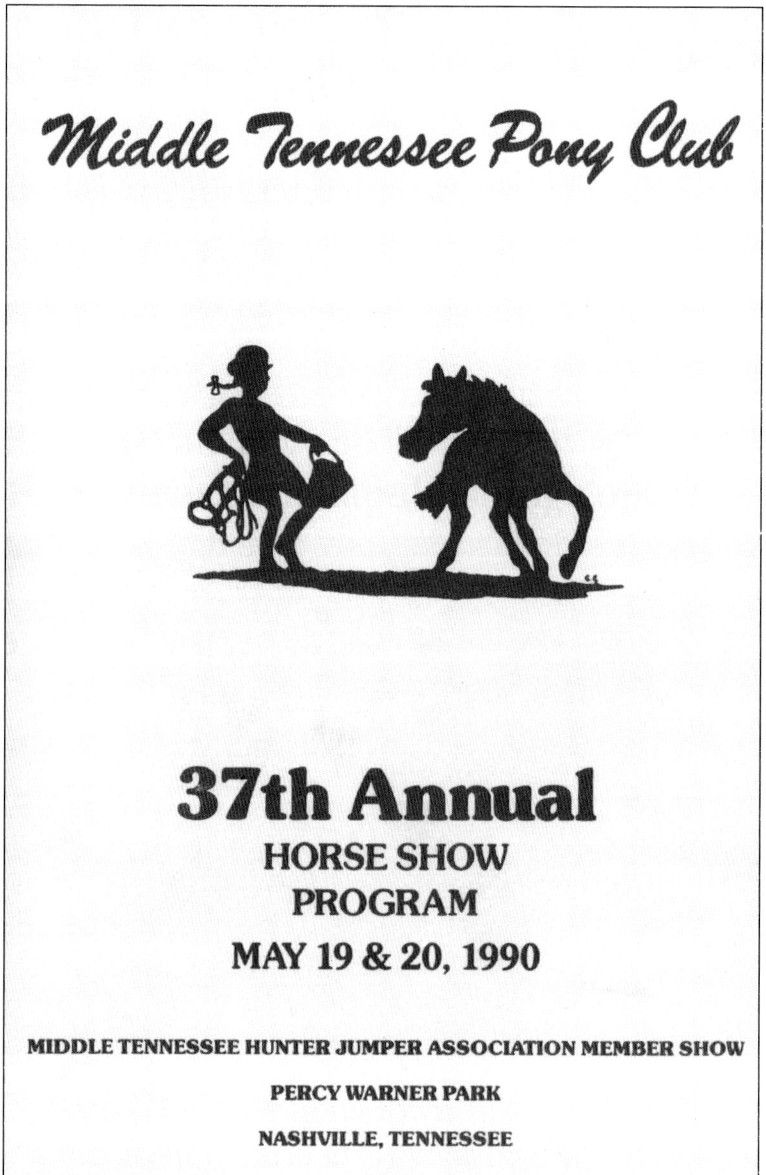

Middle Tennessee Pony Club

37th Annual
HORSE SHOW
PROGRAM
MAY 19 & 20, 1990

MIDDLE TENNESSEE HUNTER JUMPER ASSOCIATION MEMBER SHOW
PERCY WARNER PARK
NASHVILLE, TENNESSEE

The program of the 37th annual Middle Tennessee Pony Club Horse Show, held in 1990, represents the continued growth of hunter breeding and training in the region. Nationally recognized stables of the 1980s and 1990s included Brass Lantern, Brownland Farm, and Warioto in Franklin and David Q. Wright's stable in Murfreesboro. The rapid population growth in Middle Tennessee has put increased pressure upon the older breeding farms and training stables as land has become more expensive. The large stretches of land once available for group trail rides are harder to find. Most of the numerous harness tracks that dotted the landscape have either been covered or, like the old county track in Murfreesboro, are waiting for the right offer. But perhaps the new residents, some of whom are building their homes on the former 19th-century Thoroughbred breeding farms of Kennesaw and Fairview, may be inspired to join the "horsey" set and break into a two-centuries-long tradition of horse breeding in Middle Tennessee. (Courtesy of Gore Center.)

BIBLIOGRAPHY

Akers, Dwight. *Drivers Up: The Story of American Harness Racing.* 2nd ed. New York: G. P. Putnam's Sons, 1947.

Anderson, James Douglas and Balie Peyton. *Making the American Thoroughbred, Especially in Tennessee, 1800–1845.* Norwood, MA: Plimpton Press, 1916.

Geers, Ed. *Ed Geers' Experience with the Trotters & Pacers.* Buffalo, NY: The Matthews-Northrup Company, 1901.

Hervey, John L. *Racing in America 1665–1865, Vol. 1.* New York: The Jockey Club, 1944.

———. *Racing in America 1665–1865, Vol. 2.* New York: The Jockey Club, 1944.

Houghland, Mason. *Gone Away.* Berryville, VA: Blue Ridge Press, 1934.

Jessup, Georgann and Barbara Stahura. *Tennessee Walking Horse National Celebration.* 2nd ed. Paducah, KY: Turner Publishing Company, 1996.

Lerner, Eugene M. "Southern Output and Agricultural Income, 1860–1880." *Agricultural History* 33, no. 3 (1959): 117–125.

Mackay-Smith, Alexander. *Foxhunting in North America: A Comprehensive Guide to Organized Foxhunting in the United States and Canada.* Millwood, VA: self-published, 1988.

Taylor, Louis. *The Horse America Made.* Louisville, KY: American Saddle Horse Breeders Association, 1944.

Warden, Margaret Lindsley. *The Belle Meade Plantation.* Revised by James H. Redford and Ridley Wills II. Nashville: Association for the Preservation of Tennessee Antiquities, 1988.

Wills, Ridley II. *Belle Meade Bloodlines.* Nashville: Association for the Preservation of Tennessee Antiquities, 1990.

———. *The History of Belle Meade: Mansion, Plantation, and Stud.* Nashville: Vanderbilt University Press, 1991.

Wallace, Louis D., ed. *The Horse and Its Heritage in Tennessee.* 3rd ed. Nashville: Tennessee Department of Agriculture, 1951.

Womack, Bob. *The Echo of Hoofbeats: The History of the Tennessee Walking Horse.* Shelbyville, TN: The Walking Horse Publishing Company, 1973.

Discover Thousands of Local History Books Featuring Millions of Vintage Images

Arcadia Publishing, the leading local history publisher in the United States, is committed to making history accessible and meaningful through publishing books that celebrate and preserve the heritage of America's people and places.

Find more books like this at
www.arcadiapublishing.com

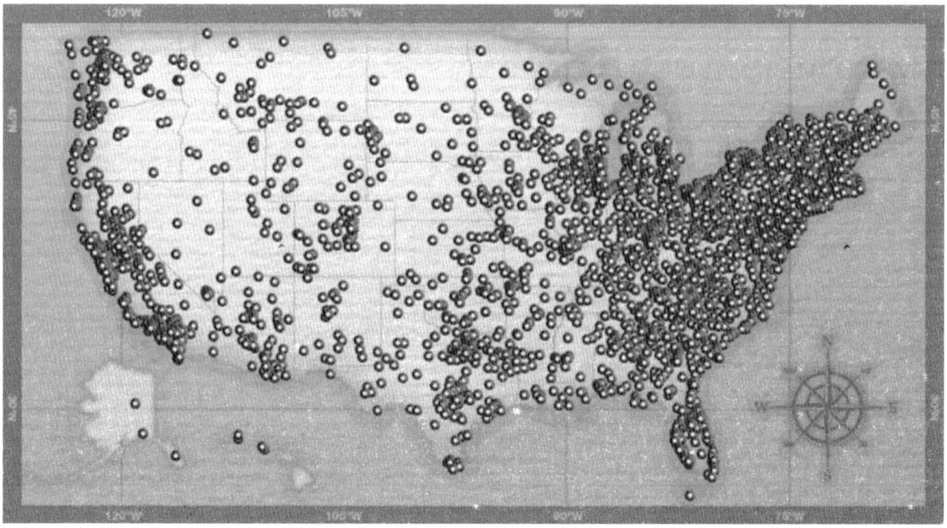

Search for your hometown history, your old stomping grounds, and even your favorite sports team.

Consistent with our mission to preserve history on a local level, this book was printed in South Carolina on American-made paper and manufactured entirely in the United States. Products carrying the accredited Forest Stewardship Council (FSC) label are printed on 100 percent FSC-certified paper.

MADE IN THE USA